Flight Quack

The true story of the Vietnam War's most decorated flight
surgeon, who became a CIA assassin

By:
Alan S. Levin, M.D., J.D.
and
J.B. Gentry

Flight Quack
The true story of the Vietnam War's most decorated flight surgeon, who became a CIA assassin

ISBN: 978-1-7346391-5-5

Phaktory
1401 Lavaca St #40458
Austin, TX 78701
contact@phaktory.com

Cover design and layout by Phaktory
https://www.phaktory.com/
Photo by Sgt. R.E. Wilson, USMC

Foreword

As always, thank you Vera for your inspiration and guidance.
To J.B. Gentry, my co-writer, I appreciate your creative input and writing skills which were instrumental in completing this project.

******

My story shocks rational senses and stirs controversy.
Just what I intended.
The debates will continue, I hope.
With a shared mission of ending proxy wars, protecting our precious resources and discovering a more peaceful and harmonious co-existence.

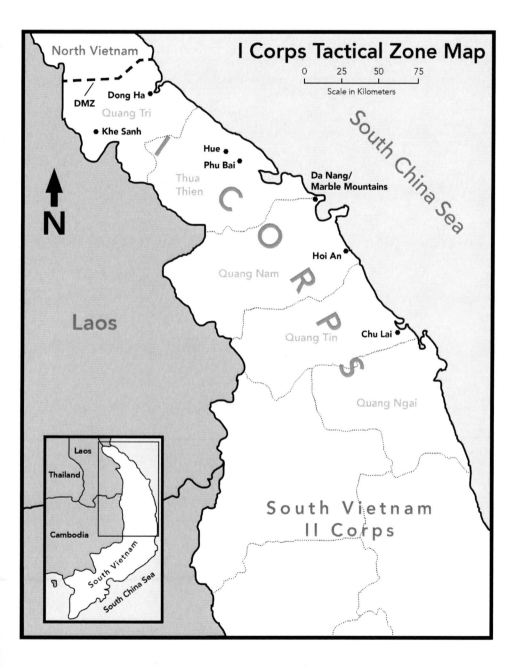

I Corps Tactical Zone Map

Scale in Kilometers
0   25   50   75

North Vietnam

DMZ

Dong Ha

Quang Tri

Khe Sanh

Hue

Phu Bai

Thua
Thien

Da Nang/
Marble Mountains

South China Sea

Hoi An

Quang Nam

Quang Tin

Chu Lai

Quang Ngai

Laos

I C O R P S

N

South Vietnam
II Corps

Laos

Thailand

Cambodia

South Vietnam

South China Sea

Table of Contents

Prologue

I became a pediatrician – a healer.

Then I got drafted, sent to the Vietnam war and was transformed into a killer.

Growing up poor in West Chicago in a family of Russian Jewish heritage, I was gifted physically and academically, graduated medical school and had completed my pediatric post-doctoral fellowship program, envisioning a career in research into the emerging medical field of immunology.

I'd taken the Hippocratic Oath and swore to "Do No Harm."

Then, in 1965, as the Vietnam War was rapidly escalating, I got a Doctor's Draft notice from the Selective Service System in my mailbox.

They got me, I knowingly admitted to myself.

At that time, most physicians were able to fulfill any military obligation by securing assignments entirely removed from the controversial far-away war in this tiny Southeast Asian nation, which for centuries has been the battleground of world powers, fueled by quests for political control, corporate profiteering and international drug trafficking.

I thought that I had accomplished just that, being assured by military recruiters I had visited of being given a Navy commission in aviation as a flight surgeon, on a potential track to astronaut training and Earth-orbiting research in immunology.

Living a life-long dream.

Flying airplanes and exploring space.

All on Uncle Sam's dime!

Going through Navy flight training was literally a blast. All the physicians in my class were aviation enthusiasts, with their plans for their military service laid out. Then, a harsh reality began to creep over us. We weren't regular Naval aviation officers. We were reservists and placing even a further stigma on us, we were (oh, yeah) draftees. Whatever we were told we'd be pursuing in the military was apparently being put on-hold. We were headed to Southeast Asia.

"Aren't doctors considered too valuable to send into actual combat?" We re-assuredly asked each other. Any anxiety over a war-time assignment was dampened significantly by the awareness that physicians caught up a war would be typically assigned to aviation bases or offshore ships away from the front lines. Unfortunately, I didn't quite fit the military mold and have always been a bit of a rebellious loud-mouth. In the past, such behavior has gotten me into trouble. And, it did so again.

While in training at the Pensacola Naval Air Station, I apparently pissed-off one of my commanding officers, who had the power to transfer my ass from the Navy into the Marines as a flight surgeon and assign me to the front lines in the Vietnam conflict. I didn't realize at the time that this meant I would probably get killed or go crazy.

I'm still alive, obviously. But, I did go insane. I admit it.

It was February of 1967 when I first landed in Dong Ha near the DMZ in Vietnam. That year Americans enjoyed the first Super Bowl game on their newly acquired color televisions. We mourned the loss of three Apollo astronauts in a launchpad capsule fire. A New Orleans prosecutor claimed to have solved the JFK assassination. The Grateful Dead and the Jimmy Hendrix Experience released their debut albums. And, hippies celebrated their Summer of Love.

Support for the war came from notable sources: Bob Hope, a Hollywood legend who entertained the troops abroad, commented "Like it or not, we've fallen heir to the job of Big Daddy to the free world," calling anti-war dissidents, "traitors." Starring in the 1968 film, "The Green Berets," John Wayne called the war "a noble cause," insisting it was "damned necessary" to stop communism.

Hundreds of thousands of young brave Americans heeded this call to duty and signed up to join the war effort, making up 2/3 of the 2.7 million who served. Seventy percent of the 58,000+ who lost their lives in the war effort were volunteers. The average age of the KIAs (Killed in Action) was 23.11 years. Sixty-one percent of them were under 21 years of age.

I watched many mortally wounded enlisted boys, as I call them,

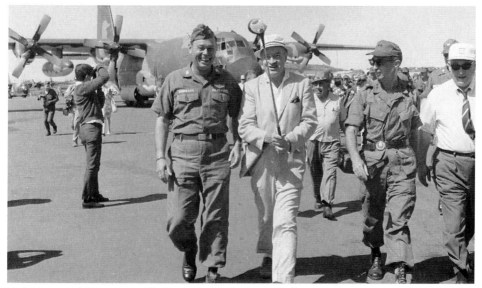

Bob Hope and his star-studded cast touch down at Pleiku Air Base in Vietnam on December 19, 1966 for his Christmas program (Credit: USAF)

volunteer or draftee, take their final breaths. On their faces – and I still remember a lot of them – I saw a son, a husband, a father or a brother.

At that time, with mounting casualties and escalating costs, resistance to the distant Vietnam War was swelling nationwide. Peace activist Dr. Martin Luther King denounced it. In Washington D.C., New York City, San Francisco and elsewhere, tens of thousands marched in protest. Boxing champion Mohamed Ali had refused military service.

Despite growing and widespread objections, throughout my tour of duty, a tremendous build-up of weaponry and military personnel was occurring on both sides of the conflict. The air and ground battles raged with greater scale and intensity. At the war's peak, America had committed enough troops to fill five major college football stadiums. LBJ told the nation that "we are making progress." General William Westmorland, Commander of the United States Forces, claimed our enemies were "certainly losing."

Were they?

During this massive escalation, enemy forces were secretly preparing for the country-wide Tet Offensive that was launched against us in January of 1968, resulting in months of ferocious fighting which inflicted heavy losses on both sides.

Although we were winning the big battles, we were not defeating

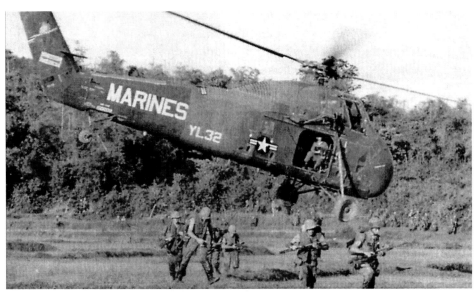

A U.S. Marines UH-34 delivers troops to the battlefield during escalation in front-line fighting (Credit: USMC)

our enemies.

Elected on the promise of ending the war, President Richard Nixon couldn't afford to "lose" it politically, and extended the conflict for years, pumping billions upon billions of dollars into training and arming the South Vietnamese military forces, to continue fighting after we pulled out. However, conflicted and corrupt, the GVN (Government of the Republic of Vietnam) and its military collapsed due to eroding public support. On April 30, 1975, with the fall of Saigon, the war was over.

Human Cost of the Vietnam War

Before America negotiated its stalemate, 211,455 U.S. service members had been killed or wounded, or about one in ten who served. The Army and Marines suffered 95% of those losses. The Army had 134,982 killed or wounded, or 63.8%. The Marines had 66,227 or 31.3% – nearly one in four.

That's not a typo, one in four.

I feared I'd be one of them. Carrying a ton of apprehension, I presented myself to my commanding officer in a noticeably fresh uniform. I was given a brief greeting and no real orientation. I was supplied with guns, body armor, basic medical supplies and ass insurance.

This is a thick metal plate to sit on during a Medevac mission, to protect you from being severely injured by enemy bullets coming through the floor of the aircraft.

When issued with all this gear, I responded –

"A gun?"

"Why do I need a gun?"

"I'm a doctor."

"Make sure you have it," I was warned, "You sure as hell might need it."

Holy shit, I thought.

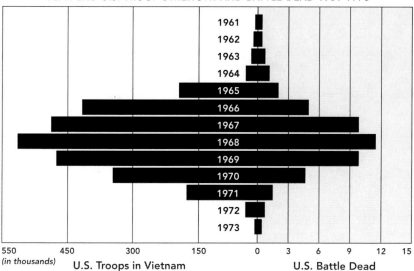

YEAR-END U.S. TROOP STRENGTH AND BATTLE DEAD 1961-1973

Utilizing Medevac helicopters more heavily in combat than ever before, the U.S. Marines fulfilled its mantra – Leave No Man Behind. Risking an aircraft and crew, we rushed to the rescue of our wounded comrades. We flew Sikorsky UH-34 and Boeing CH-46 helicopters, which were routinely dispatched into live battlefields. In a controlled crash landing under enemy fire with our machine gunners firing back, we quickly loaded the wounded. Overwhelmed with sheer terror ourselves, we practiced emergency medicine, trying to control bleeding, insert breathing tubes or establish IV lines, desperately attempting to save who we could while fighting in and out of makeshift landing zones, under the protection of our beefy Huey gunships.

During the Vietnam war, an estimated 500,000 Medevac missions were conducted. For those wounded who survived the first 24 hours, less than 1% died. Principally this was achieved through the use of helicopters. The average time from being wounded to arriving at a hospital was under an hour.

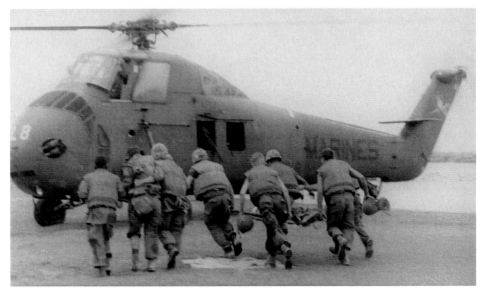

Near Dong Ha, Medevac crew members and fellow Marines carry wounded to awaiting UH-34 chopper (Credit: USMC Archives)

During my Vietnam combat experience, even though I had been sent involuntarily, I never let up while doing my duty as a U.S. Marine, working in field hospitals and flying as the medical officer aboard Medevac missions, mostly for my fellow Marines with whom I served.

However, as a doctor, witnessing the needless, senseless and brutal loss of life, I became angry and greatly disillusioned.

Many of us did.

In the spring of 1967, providing emergency medical care in what was known as the Hill Fights or the First Battle of Khe Sanh, an intense back and forth raging brawl for strategic control of Hills 881 and 861, I struggled, often in vain, to save horrifically injured soldiers, screaming in agony and disbelief that their newly-issued M-16 rifles had jammed.

They couldn't fire back. They were sitting ducks. And here they were dying, so many of them. I complained loudly after I returned only to be re-buffed. Commanding officers blamed the soldiers for not keeping their weapons clean and dry, themselves paying little attention to battle conditions in a hot, muddy and humid jungle.

Our front line bases were crudely built fortresses of airfields, bunkers and fortifications, located in lush mountains, pristine ocean shoreline and dense tropical forests, made barren from the application of toxic herbicides. We were bombarded by heavy and relentless mortar and rocket attacks, sending us diving for our bunkers in sheer terror. What our enemies blew up, we'd rebuild. Other horrors haunted us. Our base would be overrun, usually at night, with NVA and Viet Cong fighters. During my first face to face encounter, I proved to be as efficient with a knife as I was with a scalpel and willing to extinguish the enemy without hesitation or remorse. My first kill was a young NVA soldier who attacked me in my foxhole during one of their base incursions. I was either asleep or blocked the memory, but I just remember waking up with my survival knife buried deep in his lifeless chest.

It must have been automatic.
How I was trained.
Don't think.
Don't rationalize.
Just act.

Standing over the corpse of this teenager, who was trying to kill me, I boiled with fury over the needless carnage. Then, as my tour progressed, close buddies that I had gotten to know began getting killed. Mentally, I broke down completely. I developed a death wish. I wanted to die but was too afraid to take my own life.

As an effective fighter, I was recruited and joined CIA Operation Phoenix assassination teams, which were part of a broader, ongoing joint-military counter-insurgency campaign. I was throwing myself more deeply into the war and our covert operations, where we were conducting psychological warfare that strictly targeted civilians, and extended beyond the Vietnam border into neighboring countries. We were all volunteers on these missions that targeted local village leaders, who actively supported our enemies or displayed communist loyalties.

We didn't know who they were. We were directed to terminate our targets and not ask questions. We were able to do that because we had de-humanized them. To us, they were all commies and deserved to die.

Reportedly, these operations were impactful as we carried out many of them. Funding for these CIA covert activities, as I was told, came from the trafficking of heroin that was facilitated through the use of CIA Air America aircraft and flight crews. These methods reaped enormous financial profits for U.S. contractors, corrupt Southeast Asian governments, their militaries, local warlords and drug kingpins.

Apparently, the existence of a CIA-supported illicit drug trade that funded covert wars was humorous to some movie makers in Hollywood. They produced a 1990 action comedy entitled "Air America" with Mel Gibson and Robert Downey Jr., about a bromance between two CIA pilots caught up in the clandestine opiate trafficking.

Sounds like a load of belly laughs. If I saw the film, I'd probably puke.

Drug addiction rates among the U.S. troops in Vietnam were concerning, but officially downplayed. Some American vets became heroin traffickers themselves. Millions of dollars from the narcotics trade flowed into the pockets of corrupt foreign government officials, military leaders and worldwide criminal enterprises.

Additionally, the Vietnam war was quite lucrative for Wall Street as tens of billions of dollars, nearly a trillion in today's dollars, were appropriated for weaponry and infrastructure in this 10+ year proxy conflict.

In an October 1966 article in the Los Angeles Times under the headline "Economy: 1966 Best Year, Says President," Gardner Ackley, the President's chief economic adviser said, "Barring a sudden end of hostilities in Vietnam, 1967 will be as good a year for business as 1966."

On the front lines, in moments where we could let down, we sickly joked amongst ourselves, "Hey, we're not here to win this war. It's the only one they got. Make it last." At our tremendous expense in terms of human lives and suffering, huge profits were being realized both legally and otherwise.

In 1935, in his short book *War Is a Racket*, Major General Smedley D. Butler, a USMC Commanding General and the recipient of two Congressional Medals of Honor, wrote:

"WAR is a racket. It always has been. It is the only one in which the profits are reckoned in dollars and the losses in lives. It is conduct-

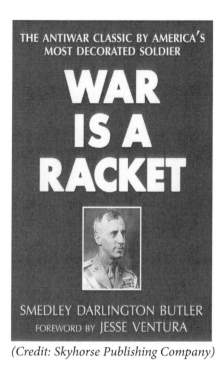

(Credit: Skyhorse Publishing Company)

ed for the benefit of the very few at the expense of the masses. Of course, it isn't put that crudely in war time. It is dressed into speeches about patriotism, love of country, and 'we must all put our shoulders to the wheel,' but the profits jump and leap and skyrocket - and are safely pocketed."

Is that really why we engage in wars overseas?

When Vietnam War vets like myself came home, we arrived to the hostility and loneliness of an America that hated us. We were spit upon. Angry protesters threw eggs on us. Within our shattered bodies and minds, we were already being tortured by the questions of why we went there. We felt profound guilt over our buddies who seemingly and needlessly lost their lives. It was as if no one understood or cared. We commonly descended into intoxicating ourselves to oblivion. In the ravages of PTSD, Post Traumatic Stress Disorder, we were tormented by nightmares, stricken with physical disabilities, fits of rage, deep depression, addiction and suicide.

Building a Life Back Home

But my story is about still being here. Drafted into the war, I was trained to treat our wounded and directed to kill our enemies. I did just that. But, I somehow emerged from that horror into a renewed life where I realized that I survived to further benefit humanity. Most of us Vietnam veterans had a lot to contribute, and we did. Like them, I felt strongly that I owed it to those guys who weren't given a chance. With Vera, my long-time partner, we built together dream careers in immunological research where we made break-through discoveries in creating vaccines, battling cancer and treating other life-threatening disorders including autoimmune disease.

I am openly admitting to the atrocities I committed in the service of my country that I dearly love and whose ideals I cherish. Soldiers aren't psychopathic killers. I wasn't. We are trained to take a life without reserve or risk losing our own. As importantly, it's all about protecting your fellow comrades. To survive, a warrior channels rage and terror into almost superhuman capabilities and endurance.

Then, even when the shooting, stabbing, bombing and bleeding stops, for many combat vets, the conflict goes on.

Over the decades of politically motivated and financially lucrative U.S. proxy wars in Korea, Vietnam, Central America, Iraq and Afghanistan, millions of us who did survive the battles were left permanently impaired physically and mentally.

Like Major General Butler, I believe wholeheartedly in the need to defend our country and protect our cherished ideals of democracy and freedom. But, I am also one of our combat veterans still standing and questioning the lasting costs of proxy warfare to our nation, primarily its youth.

Chapter One
Welcome to Hell

*"No tongue can tell, no mind conceive, no pen portray
the horrible sights I witnessed today."*
Capt. John Taggert
U.S. Army
1862

It hits you all at once, a wall of noxious odor that envelops you. You hold your breath trying not to let this vile gas into your lungs, but you can't. Mixed in this putrid mess is life-giving oxygen. Finally, you succumb, you breathe, you take in this obscene matter that stains your life forever.

Never can you forget this smell. It stays with you, always a reminder of the terrible horror of warfare. It brings back all the gut-twisting hate and fear. Of all the bodily senses, smell is most powerful in evoking memories and triggering extreme stresses on the body and mind.

The Stench

In the Vietnam war, the stench was a cacophony of smells: body odors from two or three days of sweat ripened into a pungent, musty aroma combined with the reek of unwashed feet and the peeling skin of immersion foot, known as trench foot, a non-freezing cold injury that can cause gangrene, infection, cold intolerance and pain syndromes.

Then there's the shit smell. In combat, toilet paper is a rare luxury. Even more noxious were the gut wounds that I treated, often having fecal matter oozing out. Mix-in stale urine, where a simple pit stop could cost your life. Add dried blood, gun powder, jet fuel, and aircraft motor oil fumes. All of that gets occasionally mixed with vomit from the wounded and the acrid odor of the freshly dead, or even worse, burned human flesh.

1

It's been a long time, over fifty years.
I'd like to forget it.
I can't.
It never goes away.

The Roar

WHOP-WHOP-WHOP

We're heading out to the deafening whirl of the chopper's huge rotors and roaring engines with the uncertainly of ever returning. We're Medevacs and combat soldiers, automatons, with steeled chins, loaded weapons, medical supply bags, labored breaths and secretly quivering hearts.

This time we're flying over a dense, humid rain forest about forty feet above the terrain below. Yelling over the din of the chopper, the crew chief leans over to me and shouts:

"Emergency job. Got a grunt with a bad gut wound. Might get a little hot, so be prepared."

"Okay," I shout back and reach for my equipment. An emergency Medevac means we're going in for a Marine too badly wounded to survive until combat activity cools down. We know we'll draw fire going in and coming out. We don't hesitate. In *The End of the Line*, author Robert Pisor states, "Removing wounded comrades from the field of fire is a Marine Corps tradition more sacred than life."

Preparing for arrival, I check my sidearm, the old .38 special. It's loaded and at the ready. I check my M-14 rifle, loaded and close at hand, just in case we have to fight once grounded, while loading wounded or during departure. Saving your own ass is paramount – and that of your comrades. So, I strategically place all of my medical paraphernalia around me, ready for anything that happens.

Practicing Combat Emergency Medicine

Swiftly maneuvering on approach to the landing zone, corkscrewing and falling like a rock out of the sky, the chopper begins to heave and sway. I hear the shift in the engine's power changing, signaling that we're going in. Double checking everything, I want to be prepared for my patients. In the practice of combat medical care, treating the wounded, my first job is to be sure his path for breathing is open. I break out my package of airways – S-shaped, flattened plastic tubes that go in the mouth to keep him from swallowing his tongue. I leave the remaining airways laying on the floor, in case I need them quickly.

Next, I have to make sure my grunt doesn't bleed out on me. We don't carry blood on the chopper. It wouldn't do any good anyway because we can't type and cross match. Instead, we carry plasma expanders like IV fluids and human serum albumin. I myself carry albumin because it seems to work much better. I rarely run into trouble using albumin causing hypovolemic shock, where I've lost a couple of guys using Ringer's Lactate – saline with phosphate buffers. On the severely wounded, it became my habit to start running albumin whether they looked like they needed it or not.

Doc, remember the deadly mistake? – Complacency! I'd constantly remind myself.

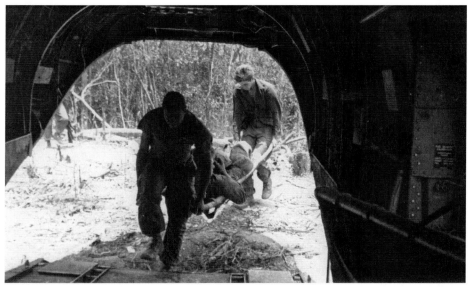

With their elite known as Devil Docs, USMC Corpsmen rush a wounded solider aboard a Medevac helicopter (Credit: USMC)

Hitting the ground, a Marine grunt was rushed on-board who had suffered a gut wound. He looked stable. He sat smiling and jabbering on the floor of the chopper as it shuddered and rose out of the landing zone. This poor son of a bitch might have been Mr. All American at home, but here he was a cruddy heap – filthy, stinking, unshaven and covered with crusted blood. Talking up a storm, unintelligible with the roar of the engine, I figured he was stable enough to make it to Charlie Med, our field hospital, where he'd be patched up by doctors who had adequate resources.

I was able to relax a little.

Suddenly, the grunt stopped jabbering. I saw a panic come over his face. He turned white as a sheet and began heaving. The constant shaking caused by helicopter's vibration must have dislodged a clot in a major arterial tear in the gut or retroperitoneal space.

The dude's bleeding out, right in front of my face!

I needed to do something. As he writhed in agony on the floor, retching his guts out and passing stool at the same time, I frantically set up an IV bottle and tubing with a needle. I grabbed his arm and started jabbing for a vein with the needle.

Nothing in the arm! Nothing in the hand!

His heart started fibrillating, his pulse became weak and thready, and he went limp in my arms.

"Doc! We're losing him!" screamed the gunner.

"No veins!" I shouted back. "No fuckin' veins!"

Shit!

There's no way we can push plasma expanders into this poor bastard now!

His whole circulatory system's collapsed!

"Can't you do anything? Doc! Do something! Do something!"

I've got to find a fucking vein! Got to find a vein!

Frantically, I searched his arms, his neck, anywhere for veins. I must get IV fluids into him. Then I panicked. A cutdown, or superficial incision into a vessel, would be damn near impossible in this shuddering shitbird. But, a cutdown was our only chance. I reached into my Unit 1 and fumbled around for a scalpel. Frenetically, I slashed at his arms, then at his neck.

No veins!

In the dim light, I couldn't make out anything that looked like a vein. I pulled out my survival knife and cut away his trousers to see whether I could find a femoral vein. Loose, foul smelling stool oozed out of the tear in his pants. I became nauseated. It was all I could do to keep from vomiting on the poor guy. I wiped the shit away and cut at his femoral regions, frantically trying to find a vein. I blindly jabbed the IV needle into the region where I hoped the femoral vein would be.

Nothing.

I cut and jabbed, jabbed and cut.

No veins!

I can't find a vein!

Nowhere!

Gradually – it seemed an eternity in that hot, grimy hellhole in the sky – the blood oozing from the wounds I'd inflicted stopped.

"He's gone," I told the gunner. "We lost him – I lost him – I blew it."

He looked at me, his eyes welling with tears. I felt tears rolling down my own cheeks.

"That's okay, Doc. You did all you could. That's okay."

Turning to the window, this tough, combat-hardened Marine pounded his fist on the M-60 machine gun and shouted to the air. "Fuckin' war! Fuckin' war! Fuckin' war!"

I'm aching all over and totally depleted. My mind is fried. I curl up on the floor in the rotten odor of the helicopter and barf my guts out.

Chapter Two

Growing Up Tough

"When you're poor, you grow up fast."
Billy Holiday
Musician

How did this happen? How did a guy like me, a Harvard-trained pediatrician, get snatched out of my rewarding life and dumped in the holocaust on the front lines of the Vietnam war? That's an easy answer. I was foolish, adventure-seeking and naïve.

Back then, the world was feverishly caught up in the Cold War. We'd fought the North Korean invasion to a stalemate. Simultaneously, we were witnessing Communist incursions in Southeast Asia. In our own back yard, the Soviet Union had attempted to install ballistic missiles in Cuba. That move created an intense stand-off between global superpowers with nuclear capability. Everyone was terrified by the image of a mushroom cloud. In our schools, we conducted drills where the children quickly hid under desks, in event of a nuclear missile attack.

How silly it appears now in the archive images, the kids crouching under flimsy school furniture, as if that would protect them.

Fear the Domino Effect

Our U.S. Presidents, the elephants and donkeys, implored that we must fight the spread of communism with military force, if necessary, and no matter the cost. They warned of the "domino effect" whereby nation by nation would fall into the clutches of this global scourge on mankind and present a growing threat to freedom worldwide. We believed them – perhaps, ignorantly.

"The United States cannot afford further retreat in Asia."
Vice-President Richard M. Nixon
1954

"I am not going to lose Vietnam."
President John F. Kennedy
Interview with Walter Cronkite
1963

"It's silly talking about how many years we will have to spend in the jungles of Vietnam when we could pave the whole country and put parking stripes on it and still be home for Christmas."
Ronald Reagan
California Gubernatorial Candidate
1965

"We do not want an expanding struggle with consequences that no one can foresee, nor will we bluster or bully or flaunt our power. But we will not surrender, and we will not retreat."
President Lyndon B. Johnson
1965

Calling All Doctors

The military needs doctors to fight its wars. We had our own special draft. And Uncle Sam got me. For those few physicians cast into actual combat, we were forever traumatized like the grunts dying around us. We witnessed the butchery, the maiming, the extreme anguish and pain. In the Vietnam war, we felt expendable in the ravenous quest for global political power and corporate profit.

So much seemed so senseless.

Our lives, as we knew them, were decimated.

My attitude?

Go to hell!

Except, I was the one actually there.

Scrappy Kid from West Chicago

I was born in Chicago on January 12, 1938, to Rebecca Ruth (Betty) and John Bernard (Jack) Levin. My father's family came from Minsk, Belarus. However, my family considered itself Russian. My great-grandfather left that region to avoid the draft in the Russo-Japanese war. He was smart – one hell of a lot smarter than me!

My grandparents, Phillip and Rosie, immigrated to America with their family, going to Scotland first, then arriving at Ellis Island in New

York before finally locating in Chicago. Rosie was wealthy. Phillip had been a Professor of Astronomy at the University of Minsk. But as Jews, they were threatened with their lives and told to leave.

They left.

In the U.S., my family did well financially. Among the newly constructed office buildings and retail stores downtown, they owned some stockyards that were located in the vicinity. Not liking idleness, my grandfather became the Jewish tailor to the neighborhoods in our area. Life was comfortable.

Loss of Wealth in Great Depression

In the first days of the Great Depression following the 1929 stock market crash, my grandparents lost all of their cash, amounting to eighty thousand dollars. For the times, this was an impressive amount of money.

Strong and resolute nevertheless, my grandmother opened Rosie's Fish Store to support the family, while my grandfather, having suffered a heart attack, remained at home. We were living on the West Side with its rough and tumble ethnic area, a microcosm of diversity with densely populated inner-city businesses and working-class neighborhoods, a polyglot of thirty languages being spoken.

The Levin family was poor and remained so.

My grandmother was big and strong, but lean. Her fish store was legendary in this Jewish ghetto neighborhood. Asked why she readily paid for protection from the local mafioso, Rosie always said goodfellas were reliable and forthright, complaining that the local police were a bunch of bullies and thieves.

The Levins had been devastated by their rapid financial decline. My parents, Jack and Betty, were no different. We all suffered. My father always worried about money. He never earned more than six thousand dollars a year in his entire life, and yet, when I took over his estate years later, it was worth a quarter of a million dollars.

He would walk miles to save a dime.

Jack was a strange, tough man with a volatile temper who was known for his prowess in the streets. He screamed, he hollered all the time. But he was never abusive to us. Not once did he lay a hand on any of us.

Betty came from a Jewish family of Eastern Russians. Her father was an engineer. During the Russo-Japanese war, he served as a Cossack Calvary officer – one of the few Jewish men to do so. Her mother was an Asian Jew, a Mongolian much like the Koreans and the Japanese. Her family owned a large fruit farm on the outskirts of Vladivostok in the Russian steppes. They prospered until Jews became personae non gratae and the family was forced to leave Russia or suffer death in the pogroms.

In 1936, my brother Don was born. I came along two years later. My dad tried to work multiple jobs, as a printer for the local newspaper publisher and for a motor club. You couldn't have more than one job during the depression, so once he was caught doing that, he lost one of them. As a family, we really struggled. We re-located to the West Side ghetto, to be near my grandparents and the fish store.

Parents in that generation were often emotionally distant from their children. But mine were good to Donny and me. I remember them going without food to properly nourish us. Imagine two growing boys, how much we could chow down. They'd starve themselves. My mother actually became anemic and fainted once, because she wasn't eating enough. My poor father would put newspapers under his shirt because he thought he couldn't afford a winter coat for himself.

They always provided for us. They'd even talk adamantly to my brother and me about *when* rather than *if* we boys went to college. Looking back at those times, I can now appreciate how destitute we were, but somehow, Donny and I never knew it. I remember living in our three-flat tenement thinking we were "upper middle class." I had it all figured out – the lower class threw their garbage out of the front and back windows, the middle class only out of the back window. And, the upper middle class? Folks of privilege had garbage cans, and the super-wealthy not only used garbage cans but also had green grass in front of their houses.

Surviving Ghetto Life

When my brother and I were youngsters, my father was extremely protective. Growing up in the ghetto of Chicago was rough and tumble. Kids got beat up regularly. To be sure that nobody hurt us until we were old enough to defend ourselves, Dad watched us like a hawk while we played in the streets and nearby parks. Many times, he would intervene in a scuffle until we could hold our own with the neighborhood ruffians.

We had a dog I loved. His name was Boy, a German Shepherd/ Great Dane mix. Oh yeah, he was intimidating and aggressive if anyone came after us. But Boy wasn't always around. And the time came when I ran to my father after being threatened by a boy who hated Jews and wanted to hurt me. My father looked at me sadly and said, "Son, you are now old enough to defend yourself, I will not be around forever. I can't help you anymore." Somehow, I didn't feel betrayed. Somehow, I understood why he was abandoning me. As a result of that, I became a survivor.

In my life, I've never lost a fight.

Within the indigence of the ghetto, gangland hoodlums were seen as heroes and attracted lots of followers. While I was able to hold my own, I stayed away from a life of crime, even though I was boyishly mischievous. Consequently, I had a somewhat lonely existence. I wasn't fitting in. No one saw me as really anything. Certainly, no one ever recognized that I might have ever possessed a modicum of intelligence or potential at anything of significance.

Somehow Making It to College

I was suspended five times from high school, that I remember. I pranked teachers. I was disruptive. If I wasn't failed, then probably, no one was. I still remember my principal who called me aside and said, "Levin, I am going to pass you, but you're a lousy student. Are you going to college?"

"Yes, sir."

He then gave me a bit of serious advice: "Don't. You'll flunk out."

Realizing My Potential

In those days, the University of Illinois accepted all high school graduates, whatever their grades. Rumor had it that eighty-five percent flunked out in the first two years. My parents had always demanded I go to college, come hell or high water. There was zero doubt. How they thought we would afford it, I couldn't have known.

Their persistent prodding led to my entry to the University of Illinois Champaign-Urbana. I fully expected to flunk out. However, this was the first real college campus I'd ever seen. That fall, as the air got crisp and the vibrant colors of turning leaves burst forth, all of the fresh warm faces I encountered appeared bright and clean.

For a ghetto kid, it was a blissful paradise. To support myself, I needed to work. What type of job would a college guy like to land? How about a cook at a sorority house? Oh, I didn't have a clue what to do. I learned as I went. Somehow, I managed to mitigate a few culinary disasters, by perfecting my Chili Con Carne recipe which delighted many taste buds.

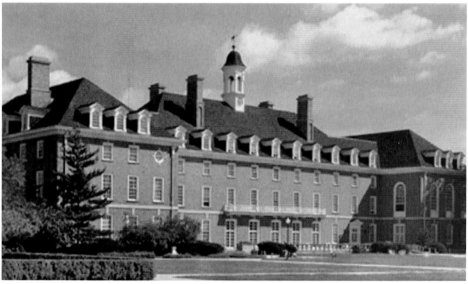

View of the Illini Union on the campus of the University of Illinois Champaign-Urbana (Credit: publish.illinois.edu)

Life-Long Colleague and Friend

Through the years and until today, I've had a great colleague and friend. His name is Sheldon Kabaker. We were roommates in college and then in medical school. We were both excellent students but also great kidders who got a few devious kicks playing practical jokes on our classmates. For instance, in medical school though everybody knew Shelly and I were smart, they also knew we were highly competent screwups, always filled with craziness, laughter and having wild parties.

Before exams, other members of the class would look to us for little pearls – everybody wanted to hear what we had to say, to know how we were able to do as well as we did. Knowing that, Shelly and I would get in the elevator and carry on, amusing ourselves by exchanging what sounded like a troubling dialog for our fellow students wedged in between us to overhear. On our way to a pathology exam, Shelly raised his voice: "Goddamn, I forgot! What was the incidence of sarcoidosis in the Swiss Army recruits in 1936?"

With absolutely no hint of anything but seriousness in my expression, I responded, "Zero point six percent." All of the others in the elevator mentally crapped – they thought they'd missed something. They hadn't.

We lived in a ramshackle low-rent house on Almond Street in the Chicago slums. In our midst were a number of youth gangs, the Taylor Lords being the toughest and most notorious in our area. They befriended us, though, which prompted us to start our own.

We called ourselves the Almond Joys.

Academic Super-Star

At the University of Illinois Champaign-Urbana, I kicked ass, completing my pre-med degree, my medical degree and a Master's degree in biochemistry. My thesis was focused on the effects of cirrhosis of the liver on albumin and gamma globulin metabolism in rats. Although my lab rats died in the first year of my research, the Federal Government continued supplying our project with the quite intoxicating Gold Bond pure ethyl alcohol for the next two years. Obviously, the rats didn't get it. No need to stockpile it, right? So, on campus our apartment became famous, or infamous, for its wild Saturday night parties, in particular for the Missionary's Downfall, or M.D. for short, a variation of the fancy drinks served at Chicago's own Trader Vic's in the Palmer House.

But instead of rum, my custom recipe consisted of ethyl alcohol… with grape juice.

I'm sorry, did I just slur that?

Working as a Cabbie

Being quite poor, I needed work. As a cabbie, my early ghetto training came to good use. Driving for Yellow Cab for several years, I shuttled fares around the city while studying medicine in the driver's seat during any down time.

Back in 1907, Yellow Cab was started by John Hertz, a Chicago automobile salesman, transforming used cars into taxicabs. He painted them yellow to attract the attention of would-be customers.

Now, part of being a good cabbie in the Windy City involves knowing where to locate all of the whorehouses and numbers rackets in your area. It must have been disconcerting though for horny johns, just into Chicago for a good time, to pile into a cab whose front seat was loaded with textbooks on biochemistry, physiology and pharmacology.

Sometimes, the guys were actually too embarrassed to ask for the local brothels.

"Where to?" I'd ask as they loaded into the back seat.

"Uh, uhm… d'ya know any good restaurants around here?" would be the response from a drunken sailor I'd just picked up in front of a local greasy spoon.

"Whaddya wanna eat?" I'd say in my best Chicago ghettoese.

"Ya know… ya know what I want," he'd say, relieved to know he was with a peer.

"Sure. How much do you want to spend?"

And off we'd go.

M.D. with Honors

All of those front seat study sessions paid off. I got my M.D. degree with honors – Alpha Omega Alpha. From there, the doors swung open at a couple of premier training programs. I could have gone to Stanford with the more laid-back California atmosphere and cool climate. In Boston, on the other hand, the Harvard program was a hard-nosed Yankee affair, charging at full speed, while enduring hot, humid New England summers and withstanding the furiously frigid winter snowstorms.

Excuse me, I'm from Chicago – pounded by the "Hawk" off Lake

Michigan. As Lou Rawls sings in Dead End Street, "That wind not only socks it to you, it socks it through you, like a giant razor blade rolling down the street."

Moving to Boston, I'd chosen Harvard, completing a Pre-Doctoral Fellowship in Pediatric Immunology.

My Wife to Be

Despite the rigors of medical school with my research and the pediatric fellowship, I took it on like a happy-go-lucky young man facing one exciting adventure after another. That included falling in love. Her name was Pam Bakus, this gorgeous gal I met during my junior year in medical school. She was from Harvard, Illinois, a small diary-farming town. She was a junior in nursing school.

Besides having a nice personality, she was quite lovely – and to me, easily the nicest legs at the University of Illinois. Yes, I had the hots for her, but came to genuinely appreciate her for how bright she was. We fell in together and while I was at the highly-rated Boston Children's Hospital, Pam worked as an R.N. at the Veterans Administration, contributing significantly to meeting our household expenses.

Enraptured with the dream of lucrative careers and a big family, we married and were planning to have a lot of children.

Restless for Adventure

Although in the eyes of others I had become quite a success, believe it or not, I still felt I had somehow failed myself. I'd busted my butt, totally putting aside all of my own adventurous dreams. I'd failed to fly airplanes, to explore and to wander. I craved daring life experiences, not just laboratories, hospitals, clinics and classrooms. Everyone told me, "It's crazy to do what you want to do. Don't be a naive child. Do what we say, get on the right track and enjoy the ride." Well, I'd cruised down that track in their wise opinion – the mainline, nonstop to success, security, position, responsibility and respect.

Me? I was bored and wanted more.

I was a fool.

Chapter Three
Want to Be an Astronaut?

*"Do the impossible, because almost everyone has told me
my ideas are merely fantasies."*
Howard Hughes
Hughes Aircraft Company

This is a chance of a lifetime!

Yes, I believed them. When I responded to my military doctor's draft notice, I readily accepted the U.S. Navy recruiter's assurances – become a naval aviator and fly into space. Wow! Here they were delivering me from my mundane life. I would soar into the skies. Plus, I was avoiding the Army, where plenty of doctor draftees were ending up.

What a deal! They told me.

You'll be a Naval officer.

Get your wings.

Become an astronaut, doing medical research in space.

It's all on us!

Not Regular Just Reserve

In reality, I was just a reservist, a draftee, not a regular commissioned officer. When my Harvard fellowship came to a conclusion, as part of the Doctor's Draft, they could do whatever they wanted with me. Like every male medical student in this country, the Selective Service had tracked my ass and, without an exemption, was requiring me to show up. However, I did have a choice – either enlist in the Army or take a commission in the medical corps of any branch of the service.

Naval aviator and flight surgeon! rang mightily in my mind.

Pam and I were excited. We shouldn't have been. Oh, I got to fly and go to distant places. Not why I thought I would. Definitely not how I had thought.

At that time, the both of us shared quite conventional goals and ambitions. We wanted careers and to raise our kids in a rural area with access to jobs at a major medical center. Our life in Boston seemed to me ideal, but Pam really didn't enjoy it there. I was gone all the time with my demands at the hospital. Often, my schedule consisted of working thirty-six of every forty-eight hours. She was a lonely new-lywed and not happy about it.

As a consequence, my draft notice actually brought some relief for her. Landing on the U.S. Government's payroll meant a good income for us and leisure time for her. Thus, she was really positive and supportive about my potential military career path and the lifetime benefits it provided. In those days, military service paid off, building a secure future for you and your family. Even in the event physicians were called up during a war, they were rarely, if ever, involved in combat operations.

I lost that bet.

When I got drafted, it was the farthest thing from my mind that over a 12-month period of my young life, I would ever be exposed to ongoing, terrifying, gut-wrenching, life and death battles, that would constantly threaten my life, driving me insane and re-shaping who I was.

I could have avoided that. I didn't.

Safe but Boring Path

Initially, when I showed my Selective Service invitation to Dr. Fred Rosen, my boss, a well-renowned Harvard pediatric immunologist and superb clinical investigator, he exclaimed, "Oh my God. We're going to have to do something about this! We've got to think about your career. You just can't go into the Army! Right now, I want you to go to the National Institutes of Health and interview with Dr. Sheldon Cohen about taking a NIH fellowship. That should satisfy your Selective Service obligation. Just in case that doesn't work, I also want you to go to Walter Reed Army Hospital and talk to Dr. Elmer Becker – he's a colonel in the Army, and he runs a first-class immunological research lab. At least, if you have to go into the military, you can just continue your work there."

Dr. Rosen had it all figured out. He was going to get me out of the draft. He was going to pull strings and use his connections to liberate me so that I could continue my promising career in immunological research.

I should have been happy. I wasn't.

Again, someone else was laying out my future for me. But I dutifully went from Boston to Washington, D.C., for interviews with the people who were going to enable me to avoid the war and allow me to serve my country by doing medical research.

I met with Dr. Cohen and discussed taking a commission in the Public Health Service. That same day, I went to Walter Reed Hospital to talk about joining the Army and doing immunological research with Dr. Becker in his Special Immunology Laboratory housed in the basement of the hospital.

Just the idea of spending two years of my life doing immunological research in the bowels of that building put me in the doldrums. I remember climbing out of that windowless warren of rooms into the bright sunlight under a brilliant blue sky. As I walked along, a sign, literally, was given to me. On a Chrysler convertible driving by, painted on the side, I saw the iconic image of large gold United States Naval Aviator wings, along with the message, "Fly Navy."

That's it!

I'm going to go to flight school!

The war's ending I hear. I'll never wind up there.

Joining Navy a Family Tradition

My brother Don and I are certainly quite different. He sought all of the trappings – business success, fancy cars and fine clothes. I wanted adrenaline, pure and simple. Like our father before him, Don had chosen the Navy. Now, so would I.

To avoid getting drafted in 1963, Don served a sedate and comfortable six months active-duty reserve at the Naval Air Station in Nashville, Tennessee. Maintaining his family's reputation, Don was always in trouble. Although he cut a fine figure, he refused to wear the uniform appropriately, refused to salute, and was disrespectful to authorities. He was, however, punctual and efficient in his job in aircraft communications. Apparently, as insolent as he was, his commanding officers nevertheless liked him.

Finally, one called him into his office and asked, "You know, Levin, you're always in trouble. How do I get you squared away?" Without a moment's hesitation Don responded, "Well, why don't you try discharging me?"

They did.

So here I was on the cusp of doing just what Dad and Donny had done. Joining the Navy seemed to be a family tradition. I guess it's where both Don and I got our deep irreverence towards military worshiping. My maternal grandfather had been a highly decorated Cossack in the Russian cavalry but because he was a Jew, he was told to leave Russia. My maternal uncles had gotten battlefield commissions and had been highly decorated heroes in the Army during World War II. They returned home to quotas for Jews in college and business. My family didn't carry a high regard for how militaries were being run. At the same time, though, there must be something in my family genes that drove us all to go into military service – and then get into trouble.

What a Gig – Spaceships or Aircraft Carriers

At the University of Illinois, all males were required to enroll in the ROTC and I joined the Air Force, due to my love of aviation. I was in the program for the obligatory four semesters, but then failed when I overslept for my final exam and missed it. I thought about dropping out of college and entering the Navy Air Cadet program. My professors, however, convinced me not to.

Now, I was an M.D. and eligible for flight training as a Navy flight surgeon. Finally, I could get my wings. From there, at best, I would be off to a Naval medical research facility and study the effect of weightlessness on the immune response while continuing to train toward being selected for the astronaut program.

At worst, I could be performing any temporary wartime service, on a secure air base in a hospital or floating off the coast somewhere on a big aircraft carrier, sleeping on clean sheets and eating three square meals a day. It sounded like a grand and brilliant plan. I seemed to be walking a bit taller and with greater ease. Either of my options in the Navy trumped being stuck in the Army or the Air Force. So, in late

1965, I marched up to Captain Weaver, the chief Naval recruiter in Washington, and identified myself.

"My name is Alan Levin and I...."

Before I'd gotten any further into my introduction, the captain interrupted, "Oh yes, you just recently graduated from the University of Illinois. Aren't you someplace in Boston now?"

All of a sudden, I felt uneasy. Did this guy know all about me? If so, he must know about most, if not all, of this year's medical school graduates. I decided to test him. "Yes, sir. Do you know where my friend Sheldon Kabaker is going for his next year of training?"

He thought for a moment. "Kabaker... Sheldon Kabaker. Oh yes, he did his internship at Letterman Army Hospital in San Francisco. He's on his way to the First Cavalry Division at Fort Benning in Columbus, Georgia. Then he's off to..." He abruptly paused, having noticeably made the decision not to finish the sentence. His response was beyond discomforting, it was frightening. Why was this guy so well-versed on all the medical school graduates? What exactly did the U.S. military have in store for us?

U.S. Military Build-Up in Vietnam

What suspicions I had, I confidently or perhaps arrogantly dismissed. They had me, I realized that. But I was in control of my future. I believed I had it made in the shade. Actually, I was in the dark, clueless to what lay ahead. While I maintained my illusions, a giant build-up of forces was underway in Vietnam on both sides of the conflict, with a huge influx in the number of troops and massive arms escalation. We were being assured that America was winning and soon it would be over.

Still concerned, I returned to the captain, re-iterating my planned course of action in the military after my training. He cautiously warned me: "Of course, we can't guarantee your billet after you finish flight school, but I promise you, I will work very hard to get you what you want."

I commenced to re-assure myself, shrugging off "can't guarantee" in my fool-hearted abandonment of reason or rationale. Like a hungry fish before a dancing lure, I swallowed his pitch and commenced the paperwork for joining the Navy program. I was eager to start. I wanted to go to flight school right then, but the good captain told me that all classes were filled. The next class that I could enter was Class 112, which started in six months. So, I signed up – joining the Reserves and for that brief period of time, carried the green Navy Reserve card identifying me as a Naval Lieutenant, without having started any assignment.

It sounded a little weird… *Lieutenant Levin, United States Naval Officer.*

Taking advantage of my Reserve officer status during this state of limbo, Pam and I would frequent the local Chelsea Naval Station Officers' Club. At the gate of the Naval base stood a spit and polish young Marine, on guard. On our first encounter with military protocols, we pulled up and had no idea what to do. The guard flagged me down, then ducked his head through the car's open window to inquire, "Do you have any identification, sir?"

"Yeah, well I guess I do."

I opened my wallet and handed him my green card. He glanced at it and suddenly jerked rigidly upright. He quickly handed the card back to me, stiffened as if somebody had shoved a steel rod up his ass, and shot his right arm up into an exacting salute. Then he stood there frozen. I sat in the driver's seat with my mouth open, shocked, wondering whether to rush out of the car and stick some kind of restraint in his mouth to keep him from swallowing his tongue. Pam's laughter snapped me back to what was happening.

"He's saluting, dummy. Salute back!"

"Oh, okay. Which hand do you use?" I asked, feeling idiotic. "The right, I think," answering myself.

Giving him my best John Wayne salute did it. His hand came sharply down to his side, remaining at stiff attention as I drove the off. Our obvious giggles as we departed embarrassed the poor grunt. After we'd driven some distance down the road, I'm sure he checked himself to make sure his fly wasn't open.

Like the Levins before me, this one would never fit in the military, oblivious to how that would impact me.

Welcome to Active Duty

Finally, the time came for active duty. I was on my path to becoming a Navy Flight Surgeon. Reporting to the Pensacola Naval Air Station, I entered the Flight Surgeon Primary Course at the Naval Aerospace Medical Institute (NAMI). I'd be earning my Naval Aviator wings including aircraft carrier qualifications. Upon completion of training, those assigned to combat aviation squadrons typically wind up on aircraft carriers or air bases with naval hospitals and clinics. Rarely are they exposed to live combat conditions.

Over New Year's of 1966, we drove down the East Coast to Pensacola Naval Air Station, home of naval aviation. I was really excited.

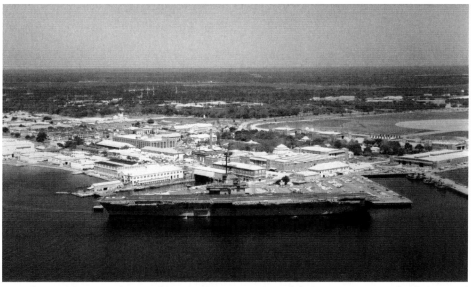

Aerial view of Pensacola Naval Air Station in 1970s with USS Lexington in the foreground (Credit: U.S. Navy National Naval Aviation Museum)

This was going to be my chance to soar into the skies. As long as I could remember, I'd always wanted to be a pilot. Every chance I got, I'd see movies about airplanes, read stories about airplanes, and dream about flying those incredible machines through the endless sky. As we arrived, we were amazed by the sights and sounds. The base was immense, sprawling in all directions with numerous airstrips, hangers, a myriad of barracks, and the airspace above filled with activity. We signed "aboard" with Warrant Officer MacNeill, a crusty old duffer with a chest covered with ribbons indicating action in World War II and Korea. He'd seen it and done it. Did he know where we were headed? Probably, but he kept that to himself.

No reason to scare us. That'd come soon enough.

"Welcome to active duty, Lieutenant Levin," he said with a peculiarly sad smile.

Shortly after, I had donned my brand new blue Naval Officer Uniform with its shiny gold buttons and braid along with white officer's hat. Looking at myself in the mirror, I was actually a little exasperated.

What a disappointment!

I look more like an usher in a movie house than a John Wayne type of military officer.

Oh, well. No movie roles for me.

At the physical, all thirty-eight members of Class 112 came together for the first time. We found out that the prior classes had approximately twelve guys in them – but all were regular Navy officers. Our particular class consisted of just two and the rest of us had been drafted as reserve Naval officers. Flight school was a plum they usually didn't offer to draftees, but America was at war and ramping up. They required more flight surgeons and they were reticent to risk the guys that might make the Navy a career, so they opened the Class 112 to the more disposable reserve officers. Unbeknownst to us, our class was primarily Vietnam-bound.

Life-Long Love of Flying

Like most youngsters, machines of mass transportation have always fascinated me. I had an elaborate set of electric trains that I played with for hours at a time. However, I especially liked airplanes. Those lofty metallic birds that carried you to far-away places – with visionaries speaking of travel through outer space. Back in Chicago in my earlier years, one of my summer jobs was as a city road maintenance worker. I was out on a truck along Edens Expressway performing manual labor on the roadway, when I looked up at this incredible sight – an airliner climbing out of O'Hare airport at the same time that a streamliner train was rolling down nearby tracks.

I was witnessing the expanding future of aviation, it thrilled me to the core.

So deep was my fascination with aircraft, I would ride my bicycle up to Glenview Naval Air Station, a trek that took three hours, just so that I could sit at the approach end of the runway under the barbed wire fence and sniff the fumes from the planes as they passed low overhead while landing.

Through my college Air Force ROTC program, I'd actually gotten a chance to finally fly on an airplane. I was given a one-hour ride in a twin-engine Beechcraft that included a brief stint in the pilot's seat, controlling the aircraft.

Being aloft simply thrilled me.

Next came a ride in an old four-engine prop DC-6 passenger plane. I'd taken a commercial sixty-dollar flight to California and back again. All I did both directions was stare out of the window at the ground below, how clean and orderly everything appeared.

Being up there, truly, I felt as free as a bird. Little did I know that this thrill would become a terror.

At that time, thanks to the Doctor's Draft, I really believed that I'd gotten my chance to fulfill a life-long dream. To me, it was a glorious experience. In pure flying, you move in numerous geometric planes. You can watch the horizon circle around your nose. You can feel gravity pull at your back and buttocks. If you turn sharply, you feel your arms weighted down until they're almost immobile, then at the top of the loop, you are totally weightless. The essence of flying is soaring. It's incredible to hear the rush of the wind, to feel you're at one with the expanse of space.

Our class was full of aviation buffs so we tended to have a natural affinity for one another. Like members of a fraternity, you help one another. You perform as a team with the pilot-in-command making the final decisions.

Becoming Officers and Gentlemen

In Pensacola, to initially earn our wings, we completed a six-week pre-flight course that provided us with the basic fundamentals of flying: classes in airmanship, aeronautical engineering, and in-depth reviews of the aircraft we'd be flying. We also had courses in counter-insurgency training and jungle survival. I didn't realize at the time how vital those skills would be to me.

Our highly skilled instructors quickly captured our respect. They required us to memorize the cockpit of the T-34B trainer so that we could identify every control, every circuit breaker, and every gauge blindfolded. We memorized all the critical speeds, altitudes, rates of climb and descent.

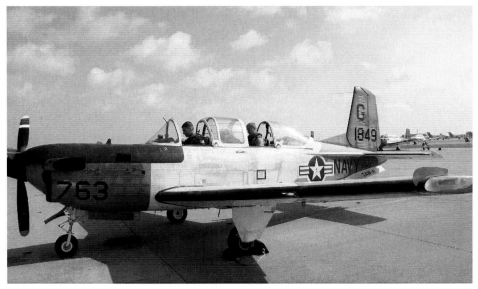

T-34 Trainer (Credit: U.S. Navy)

At the primary flight training field, Saufley Field, it was like a busy beehive, with dozens of trainer aircraft in pattern taking off and landing, all done with radio silence. Communication with the control tower was reserved for emergencies only. The rigid discipline of the pilots made the pattern predictable and safe. Learning it, however, wasn't easy. Marine Corps flight instructors prided themselves on their skillful ability to teach precision flying. On takeoff we lined up on the numbers, applied the brakes and pushed the throttle full forward, "balls to the wall." At full power we let up on the brakes and careened down the runway as inertia pressed our bodies back against our seats. We were to rotate at exactly seventy knots and climb out at exactly eight hundred feet per minute at ninety knots to an altitude of twelve hundred feet and level off. If we were off by only a relatively few feet on an altitude, we could expect a barrage of invectives over the intercom from the instructor in the back seat.

Since the instructors were fellow officers, they felt comfortable with abusive language. "You goddamn dumb motherfucker! Can't you see the fuckin' altimeter? What does it read?"

"I… I think it reads 1180 feet, sir."

"Then get us the fuck up to 1200 feet or I'll take us home and ground your ass!"

We learned how to throw the machine around in the air with precision, to dive from an altitude of exactly 5000 feet at an airspeed of exactly 180 knots – "not 175 or 185 knots, you candy-assed motherfucker!" – then snap the stick all the way back – "pull the stick to your dick" – and watch the ground disappear under the nose as we soared straight up. We'd continue straight up until we ran out of power in a hammerhead stall, then we'd kick the right rudder and pull the stick back and left to enter a precision spin. We'd line up with a road on the ground and count the number of turns, recover after two by snapping the stick forward to neutralize the rudders, raise the nose, and add power.

God forbid we'd lose more than 400 feet in the spin – if we did, we'd have to repeat, and repeat, and repeat until we got it exactly right. All primary flight training was "by the numbers." Every takeoff, every procedure, every landing had to be performed as written in the manual. Deviation was not allowed. If we didn't get it right the first time, we could expect a barrage of obscenity from the back seat and the command to repeat, and repeat, and repeat, and repeat.

For the Designated Naval Aviator candidates, these training flights constituted the initial washout period. At this point, the Navy hadn't invested a lot of money in the students, so it was a good time to select the best-qualified candidates to move onto more advanced training. For the Flight Surgeons, these initial experiences also served as an introduction to the rigors of aviation that the human body must endure.

After our primary trainer, the T-34, we graduated to a more advanced aircraft, the T-28, for further pilot training and aircraft carrier qualifications. Before stepping up, we were required to take a final T-34 flight, which was billed as an introduction to advanced aerobatics but turned out to be a full quantity of Marine Corps sadism. On this flight the instructors privately rated each other on how fast they could make their students airsick. My flight consisted of a series of wild, marginally controlled acrobatics that lasted about a half hour. I remember calling on the intercom, "I'm airsick," to which my instructor responded, "It's always good to be close to the ground when you're airsick," and began a wild hammerhead stall and spin to earth. I removed one of my flight gloves and barfed into it, hiding what had happened, so to deny my fiendish flight instructor any cheap laughs.

But whoa, Nelly! Talking about a "dyno-rrhea."

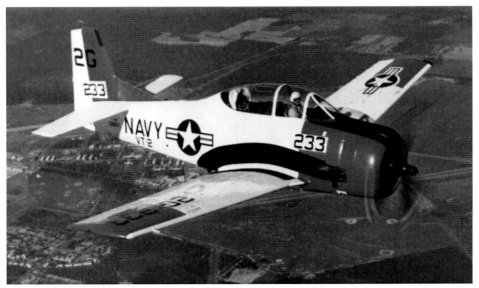

T-28 Trainer (Credit: U.S. Navy)

Aviators Pecking Order

While learning how to fly at the Aviation Training Command, I perceived a clear-cut pecking order among pilots. To become a military pilot, one had to display a reasonable level of intelligence, pass a thorough physical exam, and be able to deal with a rigorous eighteen-month training program during which approximately sixty percent of the starters wash out.

Among the survivors of that rigorous process, an unambiguous hierarchy emerges. Last in pecking order came guys who didn't get their wings but retained their interest in aviation and stayed in training to become navigators, naval flight officers, and radar intercept of-

28

ficers. These were the "guys in back" of the fighter-bombers who ran the computers and radar scopes, who monitored the operations of the aircraft in flight. They were considered "regular guys" – tolerated but never allowed into the "inner circle."

Those pilot candidates that passed through were divided into five major categories. At the bottom was the group which consisted of those who wanted to avoid combat. Usually gentle, family-oriented guys who really didn't fit the mold of the military pilot, they generally opted to migrate into big multi-engine transport aircraft. Enjoying the mobility, financial benefits, and possibility of early retirement, they often used their military training to prepare for careers in the airlines.

The remaining four levels involved combat modes: Medevac helicopter missions, tactical ground support, long-range bombers and jet fighters with air-to-surface missiles. The pilots competed with each other in terms of who were the top dogs. A lot of the of swagger depended on which pilots were in greatest demand and delivering the most impact on the progress of any fighting – whether flying into the heat of battle to rescue fallen comrades, softening enemy targets for the grunts on the ground, dropping high-altitude bombs destroying the enemy's war-making infrastructure or maintaining crucial air superiority, where our knights of the air would reign supreme.

In the Stateside training command itself, however, the hierarchy differed, with the fighter pilots on top and bomber pilots in second position, followed by ground support pilots, with helicopter pilots at the bottom of the pile.

Fighter Pilots

Fighter pilots were the top guns. They flew the sleek and fast McDonald Douglass F-4 Phantoms and Douglas Skyhawks, to name just a couple of the military's arsenal of air power and destructive capability. This pilot was usually aloof, identifying strongly with his aircraft and its performance capabilities. While flying at four hundred knots, he was cool and collected, able to manage all sorts of emergencies. Equipped to eject out of the canopy if his airplane became disabled, he could fly wild diversionary patterns to avoid ground fire or crazy elusive patterns to avoid an enemy on his tail.

His time was spent between posh quarters with clean sheets and excellent food and the extreme speed, high G-force excitement and intensity that their flying provided. When a fighter squadron lost a pilot, it was followed by a moving tribute. One moment the pilot was healthy and happy, and the next he perished in a large orange ball of flame. The fighter pilot never saw the remains of his colleagues. It was either life and health or total incineration. As a physician, I noticed that fighter pilots usually had difficulty dealing with pain. It was not uncommon to see any one of them able to manage all sorts of combat stresses in flight, but then would faint when his blood got drawn for a routine test.

Bomber Pilots

The bomber pilots flew mammoth birds like the B-52 Stratofortress or the Douglas A-1 Skyraider dive-bomber. Their duty consisted of clean and comfortable quarters with great food and recreational time, much like an executive who travels frequently. Typically, these pilots never personally witnessed the havoc that was wreaked upon their foes below, if in fact, they were such and not friendlies hit by mistake. Dive-bomber pilots were closer to the thick of it and therefore, more vulnerable to being shot down by a rocket or anti-aircraft guns. If a bomber went down, the crew either got killed or captured; they rarely ever came back to describe what had happened.

Unlike the fighter pilots, they rarely partied, rarely bragged, and often kept to themselves in small cliques. At least subconsciously, however, most were aware of the tremendous amount of damage they inflicted, and at times on innocent civilians. Due to that, many of them seemed to have morose demeanors and from what I understand, suffer far more nervous breakdowns than pilots in other groups.

Ground Support Pilots

Ground support pilots flew the Fairchild A-10 Thunderbolt, known as the "Warthog," the Douglas AC-47 Spooky, known as Puff the Magic Dragon, and the Bell UH-1 Huey Iroquois. These gunships and attack helicopters swooped down in close proximity to the ground in order to strafe targets with automatic weapons fire, missiles, rocket and grenade launchers as well as drop napalm bombs on enemy positions and soldiers. Napalm is a sticky jelly used in these incendiary devices consisting of gasoline thickened with special soaps. The pilots of these aircraft were strong, wary men extremely adept at maneuvering high-speed, heavily weighted aircraft in low-level, turbulent environments. They often found themselves exposed to ground fire and got to see the actual combatants they were killing.

Their close air support of troops on the ground made these pilots acutely aware of battle conditions. They were heavily traumatized, especially by the guilt of having been responsible for the loss of innocent lives.

Helicopter Pilots as Second-Class Citizens

In military aviation, helicopter pilots were generally considered second-class citizens – associated with the infantry. Constantly in the middle of combat in vulnerable aircraft, they were actually remarkably adept at reacting in high stress and life-threatening conditions, while fully cognizant of the blood and gore of warfare. In fact, these brave warriors were routinely involved with the wounded, maimed, and the deceased. Typically, combat helicopter pilots were just as salty as any grunt, usually quite earthy, relating well to their crews and the combat soldiers in the battlefield.

These were the guys who always got me home alive. Just the thought of them brings tears of respect and appreciation flowing out of my eyes.

Use of Helicopters in Combat

In the Vietnam war, helicopters were used more extensively than ever before, for both combat and medical evacuations. In fact, in 1932, the U.S. Marines put the first U.S. military helicopter into use.

Advancing forward a few decades, we employed the Bell Huey UH-1, a powerful workhorse along with the Sikorsky UH-34 and the Boeing CH-46. However, the operations officers – those responsible for staging combat – often had little or no experience with helicopter operations in heavy battle conditions. In the Marine Corps, these officers, some with combat experience, others none, usually came from

31

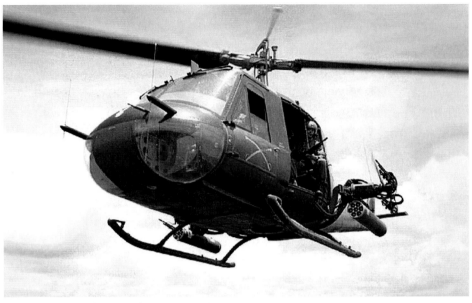

UH-1 Huey Gunship (Credit: U.S. Army)

four different groups: the air wing, infantry, armor, and logistics support. Though certainly fully cognizant of the performance capabilities of tanks and heavy artillery pieces, the officers drawn from the infantry and armor groups only had aviation experience with fixed-wing aircraft that would come in at high speed, drop their loads, and return to safe rear areas to reload.

Therefore, their combat knowledge pertained to aircraft that flew at three hundred to four hundred knots. For them, therefore, planning operations close to the ground raised issues only pertaining to weather and payloads. Because in their experience, aircraft moved far too fast to enable anyone on the ground to take a bead on them. These air wing types seldom considered the vulnerability of aircraft to small arms and more potent anti-tank weaponry.

Flying in real combat conditions, only helicopter pilots clearly understood the pertinent considerations for helicopter operation. But inasmuch as Marine helicopter pilots were second-class citizens in the pilot hierarchy, none I knew or heard about were ever invited into the operations groups, making strategic decisions that directly impacted the safety and survival of our personnel involved in ground combat operations.

There's an old saying – "If its green and says Marines, it's a tank until proven otherwise." With that mindset, the operations officers considered our helicopters just as invulnerable.

They weren't.

Designing the Safest Landing Zone

Establishing safe landing zones for Medevacs helicopters required an enormous amount of planning and execution, in the air and on the ground. The LZ site had to be identified. A perimeter had to be established. Any enemy combatants, many lying in wait, disguised or hiding in tunnels, had to be cleared out. That was accomplished by the ground forces who called us, assisted by aerial assaults. When a Medevac helicopter arrived, it was accompanied by Huey gunships and a chase plane providing that support.

Dropping into an LZ, especially when its "hot," meaning it has not been fully cleared, the Hueys would lay down barrages to kill enemy combatants or suppress them. Often, as the Medevac helicopter approached, it dropped in like a corkscrew, falling like a rock, suddenly flaring before a controlled crash landing. Often, it never actually touched down but hovered close to the ground.

Furthermore, helicopters perform best landing and taking off into the wind, in terms of stability and power management. So, in the

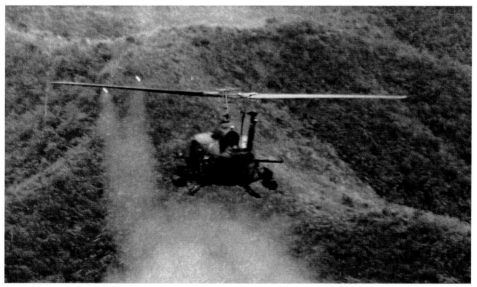

UH-I Huey Gunship fires rockets upon enemy forces during the Vietnam conflict (Credit: U.S. Army)

final moments of these maneuvers, the aircraft's movement can be predicted. Entering a combat zone, the Medevac is almost as vulnerable as a parachutist.

Careful attention must be paid to load. A chopper's carrying capability depends on outside air temperature, with their actual capacity to carry troops, ammunition, and even fuel can be more than halved by high temperatures. Overloading a bird can lead to disastrous consequences.

No, You're Going to Vietnam

Among the doctor draftees in Class 112, suspicions grew during our flight training. We realized that reservists like us were likely being sent off to the war. If that were the case, then promises made to us were obviously being put on hold. Sure, we'd been told that we could do what we wanted, that we'd be able to write our own ticket. As it turned out – that could potentially occur but only after we fulfilled our wartime duty assignment.

However, it certainly didn't involve me being exposed to any real hazard or threat to my life, or so I believed.

I am a Harvard fellow, for crying out loud.

Why throw me into a shitshow?

"Okay, no need to panic," we all re-assured ourselves. But were we just naive? Would we come back and continue on with what we had been expecting? We planned to go into surgery, psychiatry and ophthalmology, with myself looking to advance into space medical research. During my flight training, I'd actually gotten to try out the newly designed spacesuits.

"They wouldn't trash us?" We concluded. "Certainly not."

In fact, in 1965, Capt. Joseph Peter Kerwin, M.D., a U.S. Navy flight surgeon from Oak Park, Illinois became the first physician selected for the astronaut program and was a pilot on board the 1973 Skylab 2 mission, conducting science experiments. Having previously served as the NASA Mission Control's Apollo 13 Capsule Communicator, Capt. Kerwin uttered those famous words "Farewell Aquarius, and we thank you." In 1997, he was inducted into the Astronaut Hall of Fame.

I was fired up to follow him.

Still, out of concern over what we were seeing and hearing about flight surgeons going off to war, I decided to confirm that I would be continuing with my research opportunity that I was anticipating. As a fellow Harvard-trained M.D. and Ph.D., who'd been in the Navy for over thirty years, Dr. Ashton Graybiel was probably one of the most famous aviation physiologists of his time. He was among the first doctors to examine John Glenn after his flight aboard the Mercury spacecraft that had orbited Earth three times.

Dr. Graybiel, a proper, elderly gentleman, had the typical Harvard academic demeanor and proved himself extremely matter-of-fact. I came to him all bright-eyed and bushy-tailed and green behind the ears.

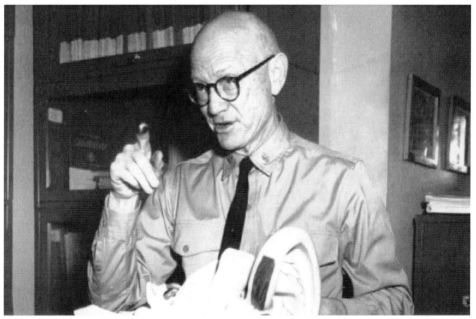

Ashton Graybiel, M.D., Director of the Naval Aerospace Medical Institute (Credit: Brandeis University)

"Hello, Dr. Graybiel. I've heard a lot about you. I'm from Harvard. I'm in Flight Surgeon Class 112, and as soon as we finish flight school I understand I'm to join your group to do research."

He looked as if he'd been blind-sided. His eyes locked on mine as he inquired, "You're here to do what?"

"My name is Levin and I'm coming from Harvard and I was told

35

that after flight school I was to enter your program to study the effect of weightlessness on immune response."

His face didn't change. He stared almost as if he were looking through me. He shifted first forward, then back in the chair. His face contorted in what to this day I take to have been anguish. He wanted to say something, but it wasn't proper. And then it came out, perhaps the first and only time he'd ever lost his cool.

Dr. Ashton Graybiel, the proper, elderly gentleman from Harvard, leaned way back in his chair and with his eyes opened to a wide ominous glare bellowed, "Do you have any idea what's in store for you?"

In my best military fashion, though somewhat shaken, I replied, "No sir, I don't."

"You're going to the Marines," he declared.

"What was that, sir?"

"You're going to Vietnam."

Can I Quit?

Hold on here! It's me, the dilettante liberal Democrat. While I had casually followed world affairs surrounding the Vietnam war, more so recently, I was far too busy being a medical student and a postdoctoral fellow to formulate any definitive perceptions or opinions.

Entering the Navy, I knew that the war was a political mess. Ho Chi Minh, the Vietnamese revolutionary, had come to the U.S. for help, but we chose to support puppet regimes under our control. Even though I was aware of the political corruption, waste of resources and human lives that ensued, before I was thrown into the conflict, the brutal realities of warfare were just like the country and culture itself – completely foreign to me.

All I really knew was that I didn't want to go.

Looking back, I see just how oblivious I was as to the terror and violent turmoil that was ahead. That's why us military reservists, lacking any real awareness, were able to even climb aboard the outbound plane. If I had truly known what would be happening, I might have chosen the stockade or a firing squad. Or, perhaps like many other draftees, a clandestine life, escaping undercover to Canada, our northern neighbor. In 1977, President Jimmy Carter pardoned those draft dodgers for their crimes. Honestly, I probably would've boarded the flight anyway. I was taught to fight.

Still pleading my case to Dr. Graybiel, I protested to him.

"But sir, I'm in the Navy."

"How old are you?" he asked.

"Twenty-nine, sir."

"You're old enough to know better. Your class is made up of draftees because it was specially selected to fill the slots in the Marine Corps squadrons that are being shipped to Vietnam. We've got a war going, you know, and the regular career military people don't want to fight. They need cannon fodder, and you draftees are it."

"Well, sir, but I joined the Navy. I'm not in the Marines."

"You are now. Surely you know that the Navy supplies the Marines with all of their medical personnel."

Those words came as a shock. I couldn't believe it. How could this happen? All I knew about the Marines I'd learned from John Wayne movies. It wasn't me. I did know that for sure. During this entire time, I had thought the worst that could happen to me would be to float off the Vietnam coast on a beautiful, clean aircraft carrier, eating three square meals a day. But now, from the sound of it, I was headed into the unimaginable.

"Sir, can I quit?"

He roared in laughter, "What do you mean, quit? They own you. The Navy owns everything you have. They own your body. They own your saliva. They own your feces. They own your urine. They tell you when to breathe and when not to breathe. For the next two and a half years, you have nothing to say about yourself."

"But, sir, I joined the Navy because they told me I could study the effect of weightlessness on immune response."

"You can. You're more than welcome in my program – after they've finished with you."

"But sir, I'm only in the Navy for two and a half years."

"Just as I said, they own you for the next two and a half years. If you want to stay in, you're more than welcome to come back to my program. I can do nothing about it."

Me, a U.S. Marine?

Me, a U.S. Marine? I was in denial. He must have been kidding. But, that's how it started – thirty-six draftees, Class 112, some to be thrust into a hellish odyssey. Originally thinking we were Navy guys, almost all of us wound up in the Marines. Most went to Vietnam. Many of us got wounded. Some got killed. Pam and I kept asking ourselves, *why is this happening to us?*

Wake-Up Call

Up to that time, we'd all sailed through training. The course work was challenging but no problem. The flying was exciting and often adrenaline-filled fun. All we ever did was study, soar through the skies and make sweet love to our wives and girlfriends. Truly, it was one of the most splendid times in my life. In Pensacola, Pam found an alcoholic rehabilitation hospital where she worked part-time, enjoying both her job and the society of the other newlyweds on the base who mostly lived in the same neighborhood.

All of the laughter ended, though. One of our close neighbors was a fighter pilot who shipped off to Vietnam and was shot down and killed. That horrible news caused panic to take root in our minds and certainly intensified our unsettledness. We'd awoken pretty fully to where we were headed. But as a training class, we distracted ourselves by focusing on earning our wings and becoming officers and gentlemen.

However, the goal of fine-tuning us into stalwart military men was a source of never-ending humor.

Never Quite Fit a U.S. Military Uniform

Our group, Class 112, was mostly Jewish. In those days, we heavily populated the medical schools, so consequently, a lot of us were drafted into military service. Although good doctors and excellent fighters, Jews show little capacity for tolerating the rigid military discipline. More accustomed to taking orders from their mothers, nice Jewish boys now faced the wrath of our burly drill instructors. Our Drill Instructor (DI), a sergeant and tough-looking tike, whose chest bristled with battle ribbons, had the harrowing task of being an enlisted man required to order officers around. Besides that, he was accustomed to working with smaller flight surgeon classes made up of Regular Navy officers who'd volunteered for military service and who respected military discipline. Despite his brash admonishments, we didn't much care about uniforms or the spit and polish appearance.

Consequently, all attempts to mold our group into well-disciplined martinets failed abysmally.

Throughout our training and, indeed, our military careers, we remained no more than a group of ragtags. Our uniforms never fit, our shoes were never polished. We tried as hard as possible not to salute. Any senior officer who attempted to mold us into the proper image of a military man we quickly branded an SOB – Senile Old Bastard.

To learn how to march and salute, we got assigned to the drill field – a large grass-covered area, complete with grandstands. Enlisted Marines always viewed our drill sessions with glee. They came to sit in the bleachers, where they took great delight in watching a bunch of officers act like clumsy buffoons. None of us could keep a straight face. All of us – as both we and our DI discovered – had at least two left feet. However, there were no laughs from him. He'd nearly bust a brain artery over having to be saddled with us.

In marching drills, we did okay – if we were only required to proceed straight ahead. We somehow managed to maintain the same direction. However, when our DI hollered out, "Colummmm Lee-eft, Harch!" what unity of motion we had achieved broke apart. No one knew exactly who went where. It quickly turned into a mounting heap of bodies. It appeared more like a drunken fraternity pool party than crisp and disciplined military drills. As always, the grunts in the bleachers greeted our clumsy blundering with loud hoots and hollers. More so than anything else, for our crusty leader, all of that boisterous commentary from the bleachers never ceased to exasperate him.

Next, came his attempts to teach us how to salute Marine Corps style, making special reference to the Navy, claiming their salute was for wimpy winnies. "Da Marines," he said, "salute wit' da upper ann at ninety degrees from da body and parallel to da ground. Da right hand snaps to da fawhed."

To afford us an example, he rigidly snapped a salute.

"Okay now, sirs, let's see a real Marine Corps salute."

Would we take it seriously?

"Ouch!" hollered Stan Lewis as he playfully punched himself in the eye.

"Cut that out!" hollered Dan Kaiser as Larry Middleton poked him in the head while clumsily attempting to salute.

After observing our bungled attempts, our DI mumbled in exasperation:

"I'm hoping none of youse assholes are some kinda doctors, sirs."

Then, came the order to pose for a class picture. We should form up, he announced, according to our rank. But none of us knew what our ranks were in relation to each other. Our DI told us to look down at the number of stripes on our sleeves. Some guys had two fat stripes, some two fat and one skinny, one had three fat stripes and one had one fat and one skinny. Who the hell knew what all that crap meant? We started asking each other how much we were getting paid. That didn't work either because some were married, some unmarried, some had reserve time, and so on.

Our DI shouted over the din of our animated discussions, "Don't youse fuckin' guys know nothin'… sirs?" Used to dealing the military's rigidness, he'd never before encountered a group of klutzy, drafted Jewish doctors.

"No, we fuckin' guys don't know nothin', so will you tell us who outranks who and we'll stand where we're supposed to," shouted Stan Lewis. Exasperated, the DI came down from the platform where he had been standing with the camera and for the next fifteen minutes tried to line us up by rank.

Finally, he gave up in disgust: "Stand anywhere you fuckin' please." So, we stood anywhere we fuckin' pleased. That was how the U.S. Navy captured Flight Surgeon Class Number 112 – highly qualified, but exasperatingly comedic.

Stan Lewis - My Best Friend

Our group was a close bunch and weathered the anxiety together, surrounded by the looming fate that appeared to be destined for us. Most of us were married, but there were a few singles. One was Dr. Stan Lewis. He had graduated from Albert Einstein University at the

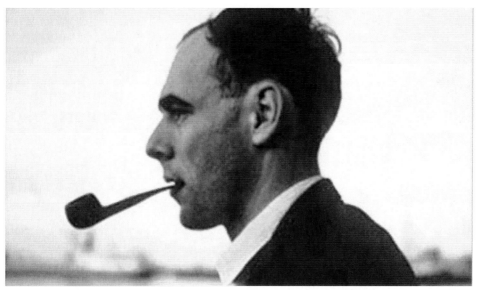

Lt. Stan Lewis M.D., my friend and fellow flight surgeon who was killed in action on January 31, 1968 during a rocket attack at the onset of the Tet Offensive (Credit: Lewis Family)

top of his 1964 class. Stan planned to go into neurophysiology, having completed an internship at Mt. Sinai Hospital in New York and having been offered a medical residency at Harvard's Peter Bent Brigham Hospital when the draft got him. Because of our similar interests and backgrounds, Stan and I became best friends.

We were both Jewish kids and we'd met as a result of our common passion for flying. Our academic interests – immunology and neurochemistry – overlapped, so we had a lot to discuss. We shared the same mentors and seemed so alike, except how we looked – tall and lanky versus short and stumpy. Stan could have been cast as a young Abraham Lincoln, with an air of distinguishment about him. We also shared a similar taste in women. Stan and Pam hit it off. I was threatened at first, but grew to appreciate the true affection that existed between us.

If anything happened to me, I knew Stan would take care of her and that comforted me.

By this time, I knew the regular navy officers disliked my attitude and I feared I was destined for trouble. The academics and flight training were not burdensome, a delight actually, but the spit and polish bullshit was just like an itch that you couldn't scratch. I was so irritated and I imagine, irritating. I always appeared a little quacky, but I was a doctor, not a military officer, so what'd you expect?

It was painfully obvious that my uniforms never fit quite right. My ties never looked correct. I did try, but never adjusted satisfactorily to the mold of a Naval Officer, as expected by the career brass. I rarely saluted anyone, and when I did, I was invariably awkward. If I didn't know what the rank of some guy was, if I couldn't remember, it just wasn't important to me.

We'll Teach You Something

As I progressed, I bumped up against, or perhaps crashed into, those ranking officers above me who took military discipline and protocol more seriously than I obviously did. Most let me slide, realizing that this wasn't my chosen calling. Others didn't and I paid dearly for it. My outward disdain for the military bullshit culminated when a Navy captain decided that none of the draftees' wives could come aboard the aircraft carrier to watch their husbands who had qualified to perform solo carrier take-offs and landings, even though it had always been a tradition for the wives of such Navy pilots in training to do so.

This was a big deal to me and I was really pissed off. Regular offi-

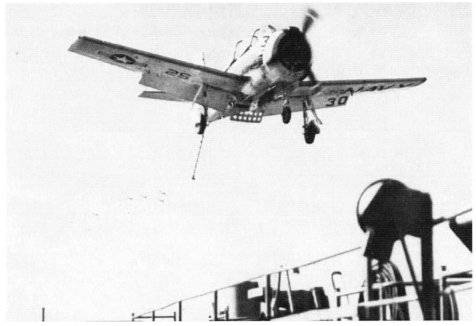

T-28 trainer landing during aircraft carrier qualifications (Credit: U.S. Navy)

cers got this privilege. Sure, I was a reserve but, goddamn it, I deserved it too. Enraged, I stormed into the Captain's office and confronted him.

"Sir, I'm Lieutenant Levin."

"I've heard a lot about you Levin. What do you want?"

"I want my wife to go aboard the Lex to watch care quals" – translated – I wanted Pam to be on the aircraft carrier USS Lexington to watch my carrier qualifications.

"I'm sorry, Lieutenant. That privilege is reserved for wives of Regular Officers only."

I could feel the hair on the back of my neck bristle. I should have smiled and turned around, but I didn't. After all, I wasn't some grunt. I was a doctor. "Listen, you senile old bastard, I'm going to Vietnam. I'm going to war. Draftee or Regular, my ass is on the line. Now you let my wife aboard or I'll personally complain to the Admiral, or the President if necessary," I shouted.

"Very well, Lieutenant," he said with a sly smile, "but we'll teach you a few things about the Navy before this is over."

I didn't know at that moment to think – *Uh oh.*

Ticket to the Front Lines

We knew that most of us were off to Vietnam. But exactly where? Being the excellent politician from New York, Stan was able to gloss over the shortcomings of these sub-humans and smile in their faces. In Vietnam, he was assigned to a single-seat fixed-wing fighter squadron in Chu Lai in Southern I Corps, a quieter area. Even better, because he was attached to a fighter squadron, he himself would never have to fly in combat.

Me, the loudmouth? I was being shipped off to the DMZ on the front lines and into battle, attached to a Marine Corps Medevac Helicopter Squadron.

I had screwed myself. I knew the brass was gunning for me. I realized they won and that I probably would not survive. Relief and comfort only came to me in believing that Stan would make it home and he could care for Pam after my death. He would return, I felt assured. Stan, the gentle giant, would marry her and provide for her.

And I would live on in their memories.

Here I was, a dead war hero in the making, a young doctor, a draftee, having risked my life and my mental health, joining rescue crews in the back of Medevac helicopters, rushing into battle to save wounded Marines, while under enemy fire. Certainly, such bravery and patriotism would be rewarded with medals, ceremonial recognition and special memorials from a grateful nation.

What I discovered was that for those of us who were thrust into the thick of battle – the chaos, brutal fighting and bloodshed – there was no glory. No music. No cheering. Only the roar of engines, gunfire, explosions and blood-curdling screaming. All that mattered was surviving. Follow your training. Kill without question or hesitation before getting killed. And, if humanly possible, bring all of your comrades back alive. However heroic, those efforts failed all too frequently.

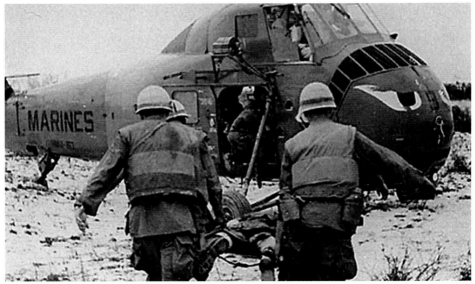

Heroic efforts by USMC Corpsmen to save the life of a wounded comrade (Credit: USMC)

With every call that comes in – Emergency Medevac! – I'd think – *Is there a corpsman available? Will they need me aboard?*

When it was "go" time, terror would shoot up my spine. My body was shocked into action. Running toward the Medevac chopper, loaded down with body armor, weapons and medical gear, I'd ask myself –

This time, will I make it back?

Will my buddies make it back?

How many mortally wounded Marines will I have to put out of

their misery?
God, I hate losing them!
They're just kids.

Shattered Under the Psychic Load

As a physician, facilitating a compassionate death in any circumstance is always a tough decision. It's done quietly and usually with the family's consent and support. Performing this act, it's necessary to separate yourself mentally and emotionally, enabling you to do what you know needs to be done. In combat, as a flight surgeon, I was routinely tasked with that responsibility. I flew on 95 Medevac missions during my tour of duty, often into raging aerial and ground battles and practiced emergency medicine on those triaged as salvageable in dimly lit bunkers under enemy attack.

In the spring of 1967, during the 881/861 Hill Fights, The First Battle of Khe Sanh, my corpsman lamented over me having to euthanize scores of our mortally wounded Marines over days of intense close-in fighting – ridge by ridge, hill to hill in steep and dense terrain.

Impossible to imagine, right? I re-live it every day. The injuries were horrific and severe. As the medical officer, I desperately tried to save who I could. I was overwhelmed at times, with a sense of helplessness, almost drowning, sinking into pure madness. We were losing so many young men with families and futures. Over and over, I was tasked, in the final painful moments of the young life of a U.S. Marine, with administering a lethal dose of morphine.

Not once, did I doubt my decision.

Mentally, it still tore me into pieces.

Chapter Four
Dumped in Dong Ha

"Older men declare war. But it is the youth that must fight and die."
Herbert Hoover
31st President of the United States

"A soldier will fight hard for a piece of colored ribbon."
Napoleon Bonaparte
French Emperor
1799

After flight training in Pensacola – that glorious, short-lived respite from the approaching hellish world of real warfare – I got transferred to El Toro Marine Corps Air Station in southern California until being shipped to Vietnam. With so much sunshine and so much flying, the Southeast Asia conflict loomed only as a menacing specter.

Still… maybe not, was the hopeful thought that Pam and I kept re-igniting.

Scuttlebutt had it that we'd win the war very soon, or that the later we got sent over, the easier our tour of duty would be. In hopes of securing one of those later tours, I traded an August 1966 rotation date for one six months later.

Six precious months more.
Surely, this damn war will be over, or almost so.
Please!

Disconcerting reports kept filtering back of flight surgeons who'd gotten wounded in helicopter Medevac operations. Nothing about any deaths. Although I normally don't panic, a wrenching anxiety kept creeping up inside of me.

What have I done? My crazy fixation on the thrills of flying just may be my undoing.
What an idiot I am.
I am goner.

47

Are the Good-byes Forever?

After my one-year tour in Vietnam, if I survived, the Navy allowed me to choose any duty station I desired for the balance of my service obligation. I arranged to be stationed at Alameda Naval Air Station in California, so that my wife Pam could live in Berkeley with relatives while I was overseas. As the end of 1966 approached, we prepared to move to Berkeley, and on a chilly overcast morning in drizzling rain we landed at the Oakland International Airport. Somehow, we knew we'd come to the end of our childhood romance and were facing a major crisis in our lives.

Not knowing is painful, made worse by the dread and anxiousness.

On yet another cloudy, rainy morning, I kissed Pam goodbye and boarded a big chartered civilian 707 passenger airliner. We all loaded in an orderly fashion, like so many innocent cattle going to slaughter, a planeload of fresh bodies that were war-bound.

Details of that trans-oceanic flight to Asia are spotty. I was so incredibly tense. We all were. I remember little except for marveling at the beauty of Mount Fuji as we descended into Japan, landing in Okinawa, where the soldiers were dispersed to their various outfits. We must have looked like stunned sheep, all droopy from the jet lag, which most of us had never experienced before. We winced foggily when our Marine leaders began shouting directions to us as we disembarked.

At Camp Roberts, a group of barracks was thrown up to temporarily house the Marines headed for their duty assignments. We were issued our combat fatigues, helmets, flak jackets and our weapons: an M-14 rifle and a revolver. For the officers, they offered a choice of handguns, either the old reliable Colt .45 or the lighter .38 special. Although handguns are not very useful in combat, the advantage of the .45 was that you could wear it in front of your crotch where it might deflect rounds that would otherwise destroy your genitals. The .38 was much lighter and smaller, with less deflective capacity, but you could carry more ammo, so that if you were stranded in the jungle, you had prolonged firepower.

I opted for the .38 special. Why? I don't know. You'd think a guy'd pay more attention to protecting the family jewels.

Spending less than twenty-four hours on Okinawa, at 0500, all the FNGs (Fucking New Guys) with their gear were herded aboard a Marine Corps C-130, a four-engine turboprop transport plane. Our next stop was Vietnam and the nasty shitshow that awaited us.

When airborne, that big bird is loud and drafty, with a pungent odor of aviation fuel and oil permeating the cabin area. We sat crammed together in hammock-like canvas seats hung from the side walls. Attached to the bulkhead hung an M-60 machine gun, for use in the event of a forced landing in hostile territory. With the only windows being little portholes in the doors, I had no view of where I was.

Outside? Probably the same chaos that I'm feeling inside.

All I really knew was this world felt completely foreign, more and more so as the minutes slowly passed.

Touching Down in Vietnam

We finally arrived at Danang Air Base around noon. They shuffled us into a large, bustling terminal building that doubled as a warehouse, with supplies and materiel stacked high on pallets in the middle of the floor and duffel bags in piles along the walls. Everything was dirty – coated with a rusty red dust that matched the local landscape.

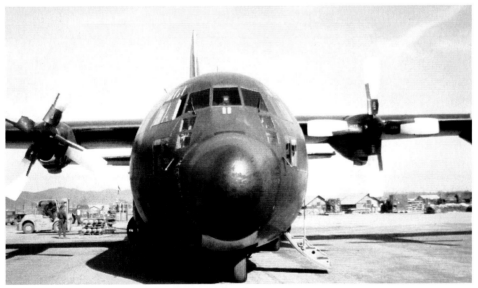

C-130 Troop Transport (Credit: Levin Archive)

Everywhere I looked I could see Marine grunts sleeping – on their duffel bags, on forklifts, curled up on the hard floor. These guys were toasted, fresh out of heavy combat and being shipped home.

Lucky bastards.

Hung on the wall, bulletin boards listed names and duty assignments. I found mine: "Levin, A. Lt (MC) USNR 689596/2105 Marble Mtn. MAG 16." There I was, my name printed in black and white.

Levin, this is as real as it gets.

My final stop?

I don't think I am walking out of here alive.

I just know it.

As a bolt of ice-cold fear shot up my back, I contemplated what battlefield medicine must be like with the deafening roar of war-time aviation surrounding me. I was headed to Marble Mountain which was the main base for all the helicopter medical evacuation squadrons in I Corps, which was the northernmost of the four tactical zones into which the military had divided the nation of South Vietnam.

I was being assigned to the HMM 265 Dragons and 361 Flying Tigers squadrons. Most of my fellow flight surgeons seemed to have non-combat-related duties so my overall anxiety about the situation for all of us was somewhat relieved.

But, not for myself.

My main base was Dong Ha, just miles from the DMZ (Demilitarized Zone), although I'd be operating out of several medical facilities in this region. Off the coast, we had access to the USS Repose, a hospital ship. In Danang was the Naval Supply Activity Station Hospital. In Phu Bai to the northwest along the coast, there was Charlie Med, a less advanced field hospital. Up in the mountains, in Khe Sanh, furthest to the northwest, we operated another medical bunker. In Dong Ha, was Alpha Med, a crudely-built clinic.

Devil Docs

In terms of Medevac missions, most of them were crewed by a pilot, co-pilot, crew chief, gunner and medical corpsmen. Like their Devil Docs, the U.S. Navy's elite medic/combatants, all corpsmen are trained to provide emergency medical treatment to wounded soldiers

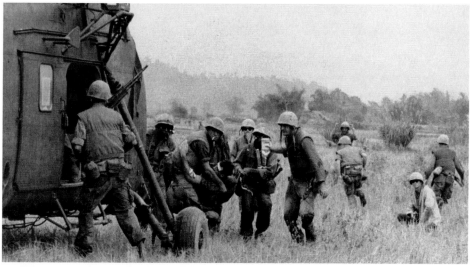
Medevac crew administering emergency treatment while loading wounded Marine aboard a UH-34 helicopter (USMC, Sgt. R.E. Wilson)

in the field, to stabilize them for transport to a military medical care facility. Their main efforts involve controlling bleeding and preventing abdominal spillage. Flight surgeons, if present, handle IVs and tracheostomies.

Typically, corpsmen complete extensive training which includes a 10-day course in Operational Emergency Medicine, an 8-week Field Medical Service School at Camp Lejeune, North Carolina and a 16-week Naval Hospital Corps School in Great Lakes, Illinois.

Way back, in the British Royal Navy, they were called Loblolly Boys, referring to the daily portion of porridge they would serve to the sick and wounded.

Knowing such well-trained medical team members would be at my side brought solace to me, but still, an intense anxiety gripped me. My chest would tighten. Breathing the acrid air was difficult and uncomfortable. Thoughts of the horrors of war raced through my mind. I was terrified.

I've got to figure a way to politick myself out of this mess!

Strategic Military Importance

In Vietnam, the DMZ stretches a mere 47 miles in width. On the front lines, along this fabricated border, the battles had been escalating. For years, both sides had skirmished back and forth, taking,

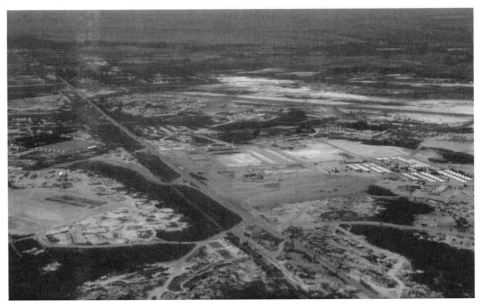

Aerial view of sprawling Danang airbase (Credit: USMC)

then losing and then re-taking what strategically was considered to be critical territory.

When I arrived in the I Corps, the Marines had firmly dug themselves in – with sprawling bases in Chu Lai, Danang/Marble Mountain, Hue/Phu Bai, Dong Ha and the outpost at Khe Sanh. Around us everywhere were the relics of the previous French occupation – the old roads, decayed bunkers and ammunition dumps. The French had fought the Vietnamese guerrilla-style underground war and gave up.

Hitching a Ride to Marble Mountain

Traveling into Marble Mountain, these rocky hills are home to Buddhist temples, ancient caves and numerous underground bunkers and interconnecting tunnels. We'd learned like the French had, that Vietnamese fighters were quite adept at concealment, and we were confronted with having to take the fight into the dark recesses of the earth, where the enemy was stationed and lurked in the darkness.

To get to the base, I hitched a ride on a large convoy truck transporting supplies.

What an eye-opener to ride through Vietnamese landscape and into the city of Danang for the first time! It bustled with diminutive Vietnamese people quickly moving hither and thither. Small mopeds with their squeaky horns could transport an entire family and their bags – a father drove, with a mother sitting behind him sidesaddle. Both would be holding a child in their laps – perhaps a baby strapped to the mom – and bags hanging off both sides. No helmets. No seeming concern or discomfort. That made me feel warm, seeing an entire family together.

How could life could ever seem this normal in a country mired in a major war that we were waging in their homeland?

Generally, the locals were not our friends, as I experienced. Most of them seemed to despise us and collaborated with the Viet Cong, but also operated as opportunistic quislings sucking off the Americans for self-aggrandizement. It was difficult to identify the enemy from non-threats among the local population. You never knew who might try to kill you – man, woman or youth.

At the Danang air terminal, as I was beginning to see as normal, red dust covered everything. Your eyes burned. Your throat became parched, followed by dry coughing and difficulty breathing. The air was mixed with smoke plus the fumes of diesel fuel and raw sewage. Humans and dogs alike often squatted to defecate ad lib in the gutters of streets lined with dealers occupying little carts filled with candy, cigarettes, lighters, and assorted touristy trinkets. Patrolling up and down

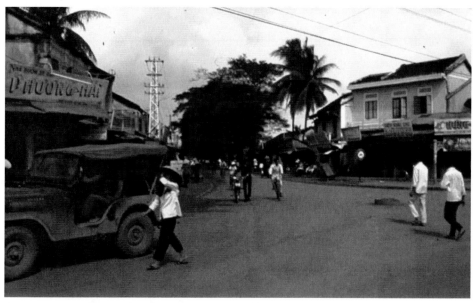

Street scene in Danang (Credit: John T. Dyer Collection)

the streets, young Vietnamese soldiers strutted about in tight-fitting fatigues, fancy sunglasses, and polished boots. These were obviously policemen and not combat soldiers.

I grew to despise those little cowards.

As my transport truck departed for Marble Mountain, we traveled through rural areas of small villages, dotted with quaint religious temples. Broad fields of tall waving rice grass and rice paddies presented a spectacle of brilliant emerald green. Heavily wrinkled old farmers drove water buffalo as they pulled their antique plows through the fertile soils.

What a bucolic sight for a war zone.

In peculiar juxtaposition to this pastoral scene, along the road stood ugly wooden observation towers, each containing allied combat soldiers who scanned every vehicle passing along the road with their machine guns loaded, cocked and ready to fire.

"Hope those guys don't have itchy trigger fingers," I joked nervously.

"Don't sweat it, Doc. You better be glad those guys are there," responded the driver. "Any one of these little gooks could drop a grenade in your lap and blow you away in a minute."

"Thanks for the encouraging note!" And with a nervous grin, I added, "Sounds like I'm gonna have a swell vacation in this tropical paradise."

Within a few minutes, we crossed a bridge over the Danang River, which was lined on both banks with small river junks bobbing in the water. Entire multi-generational families swarmed around these junks busily washing, cooking, and cleaning. I noticed a complex community of riverboats, with a flotilla of junks and swarms of people aboard.

Again I was asking myself –

How could a war be going on in such a seemingly mystical place?

Shortly, we rolled up to the barbed-wire boundary of the base. It was a sprawling, dusty outpost with barracks surrounding a single three-thousand-foot runway situated right on a beautiful, white sandy beach on the South China Sea with the sun glinting off its crystal-clear water and gentle rolling waves.

Pointing out two of the enormous rock piles, each about four hundred feet high, demarcating the beach's southern end, I turned to

the driver –

"Geez, those piles are spectacular."

"Them Marble Mountains. Real marble," he assured me. "The Buddhists think they're holy. They and have a temple carved in the rock caves. It's old, real old, like thousands of years."

"Wow! Sounds like great sight-seeing. Any of you guys go down to look at the temple?"

"Sure," he smiled wryly, "A couple of guys went down there last month. They ain't come back yet. You wanna go down to look for 'em?"

"What do you mean?" I asked in surprise.

"Them Marble Mountains is crawlin' with gooks. You don't want to be nowhere near 'em with anything less than a battalion. They're off limits unless you're crazy," he meditatively advised me.

With a hard swallow, I thought –

Not exactly your Disneyland fantasy experience.

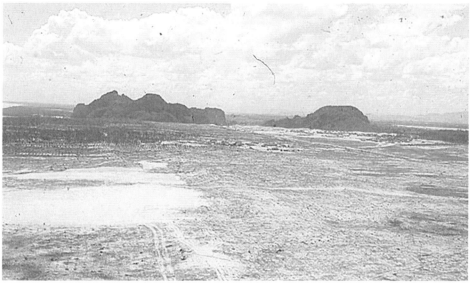

Marble Mountain from the North, taken in September 1965 by Frank Harris (Credit: USMC History Division Archives)

No way was I going to get my ass shot off sightseeing. I was going to do whatever I needed to do to stay out of the line of fire.

Or so I naively thought.

The dust-encrusted truck dropped us off at the base dispensary. I dragged my bags into this twenty by thirty-foot Korean tin edifice sitting on three-foot high stilts. The structure sported large windows covered with fly screen. There was no glass, but the holes could be closed with large shutters suspended above them, that when open, served as sunshades.

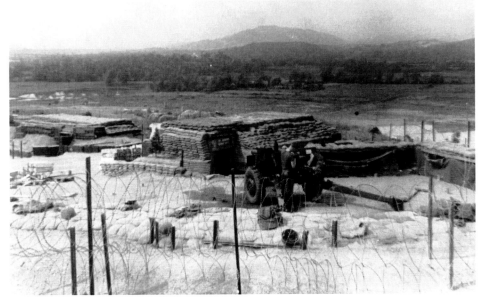

Fenced base perimeter with partially buried sandbag bunkers (Credit: USMC)

As I shortly discovered, all of the buildings at the base were similarly constructed. Entering through the front doors, I was greeted by the outstretched hand of Buddy Edrich, the senior flight surgeon on the base. He was from Class 110 and had been in-country for eleven months.

"Welcome aboard, Al. It's good to see you. How was your trip?"

"Okay, I guess, though I'm really bushed."

"Yeah, that's a hell of a trip. Nobody tells you about the jet lag. Like a Coke or an Orange soda?"

"Yeah, a Coke'll taste good about now. What's happening around here?" I asked.

"Not much. The gooks have been quiet for months. A little sporadic activity in the boonies, but nothing much to speak of." He handed me my cold drink. "We figure they're either whipped or they're tooling up for a big push. Their New Year's holiday starts soon. They call it Tet. There are rumors they plan to get active around then. So far, it looks like it's all rumor."

"Sounds like I came just at the wrong time."

"Nah, Al, don't sweat it. We've got things under control here." Dave Gillis, another Senior Flight Surgeon piped in.

I sat down on a makeshift examining table and sloshed down my beverage, when whiskey might have been better. However, I knew right away. I've got to keep my wits about me. I tried to remain calm, but there was a disquieting fear welling up inside of me that was tearing at me. It was probably not unlike treading water in the ocean, not knowing what danger might be lurking, and suddenly you see the open mouth of a great white shark coming at you out of the shadowy depths.

As the cobwebs began to clear in my head, Buddy informed me of my assignment. "Okay, Al, we've got you going with HMM 265 at Dong Ha. You'll relieve Art Lochridge."

"Where's Dong Ha?"

"Ninety miles north of here," Dave noted with a grin.

"Ninety miles!" I cried out. "That's North Vietnam."

"Not quite, genius." Dave corrected me. "It's seven miles south of the border."

"Thanks a bunch, fellows! Do you always dump on the new guy?" raising my voice in a disquieting tone. "Isn't that the job of one of you combat-hardened veterans to be up there?"

"We're short. We're going home in a couple of weeks. It's your turn in the barrel. We old timers have paid our dues," Buddy offered in a matter-of-fact fashion without expression. "Besides it's quiet up there. Nothing's happened there in months. Don't sweat it – all you'll do is fly a few priority Medevacs. They never have emergencies."

"Yeah," Dave chimed in. "If you don't look out, you could die of boredom up there."

Chopper to My New Home

"Okay. Okay." I said calming down. "How do I get there? Grab a taxi?"

"Funny, FNG!" which is what they called any newbie. Being clueless, an FNG was also considered potentially dangerous, not reacting correctly in a life and death situation. Here, Buddy was smiling broadly, telling me, "You go up there tomorrow on a resupply chopper. Let's go to the chow hall and grab some dinner. Afterwards I'll buy you a beer at the O club."

Betcha there's a lot of hitting the bottle around here, I imagined.

So off we went for my first in-country meal. Being a typical Marine Corps rear area aviation facility, Marble Mountain had pretty tasty food served cafeteria-style with long tables and benches. Given where we were, the atmosphere proved surprisingly pleasant as I chowed down on roast beef with a healthy variety of vegetables and fresh salad. For dessert, I remember having cake and ice cream. After dinner, as promised, we went to the O – for officers' – club for drinks. All of the guys appeared to be in a good mood. What brought this about was that for several weeks, there'd been little combat activity in the region.

Trying to make conservation, I somewhat nervously observed, "War is hell, ain't it."

"It can get a little hairy once in a while," Buddy replied, "but it's mostly not like that. I hope you brought a lot of good books. Your biggest enemy will be boredom."

"I can handle that," I offered, as we stumbled off to our bunks. I'd begun to feel that perhaps this tour of duty might turn out to be not so bad.

I was still trapped in my naiveté.

Guns, Knife, Unit 1 and a Cement Shirt

Morning arrived with warm and brilliant sunshine. The hustle and bustle never ceased. After breakfast as I started back to the hootch to grab my bags, Hank Gianni, the chief corpsman at Marble saw me walking past the dispensary. He came out carrying some equipment. "Hey Doc, take this cement shirt and a Unit 1 medical supply kit," he said, handing me a pair of molded plates covered with green khaki canvas. The front plate of the bulky vest was shaped to cover the chest with a separately attached skirt to cover the genitals. The other plate covered the back with another skirt to cover the rectum.

"You wear this on Medevacs. Believe me, you won't think it's too heavy, when the bullets are flying around you. They say it'll stop a 50 cal. You can detach those skirts – they're awful bulky. Nobody wears

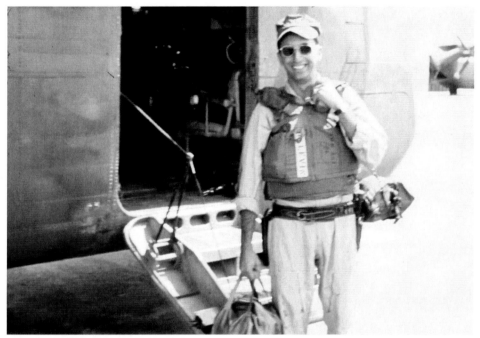

Lt. Al Levin, M.D. in front of Medevac helicopter wearing flight suit with cement shirt, medical bag, and personal weapons (Credit: Levin Archive)

them. In the Unit 1 are your medical supplies – always carry it full of everything. You never know."

"This place gets more interesting every day," I nervously joked. "Thanks for the stuff. Hope I never need this shirt."

"Need it or not, Doc, never be in a chopper without it," he warned, slapping my shoulder and ducking back into the dispensary.

Boarding the CH-46A re-supply chopper, headed for Dong Ha, I picked up my load to see just how much it weighed.

Jeez!

As it turned out, I needed all of it, as I was so forewarned – the body armor, the helmet, the medical equipment, the guns, knife and ammunition.

Everything I have right here relates to either killing or keeping from dying.

Chills ran through my spine.

Aboard my transport that day, besides the two-man crew and myself, the belly of the chopper was loaded with food and mail for the Marines at various bases in the I Corps – Gio Linh, Con Thien, Cam Lo, the Rockpile, and Khe Sanh. Once we reached cruising altitude, the co-pilot asked the gunner to plug me into the intercom so he could talk to me. "Hi, Doc. Welcome to Vietnam. I hear you're going to be the new quack at Dong Ha," came the voice over the intercom. "I'm Doug McAlister and the pilot here's Charlie Pitman."

"Hi guys, you all tour guides?"

"You'll see plenty of this route before the year's out. We call it the milk run. Our squadron flies regular resupply and mail shuttle birds. As you can see, we climbed out of Marble to the east over the beach and then out to sea. We'll get up to a five-thousand-foot altitude and a half mile out at sea. If we lose our engines, we can autorotate back to the beach from that far out. Five thousand feet over the water minimizes our exposure to small arms fire. Nothing smaller than a 50 cal can do any major damage to us here and it'd be pretty hard for the gooks to keep any anti-aircraft guns or SAM's on those junks you see down below."

Briefly pausing to check something, he continued, "Hell, it'd be damn hard for them to keep a 50 cal with ammo hidden aboard one of those dingys. You never know, though. They could get lucky with a 30 cal, but so far anyway, nobody's taken any rounds along this route, using these tactics. Sit back, relax, and take in the scenery, Doc – this is probably going to be the safest hop you'll take in-country."

"Safest as opposed to what… most dangerous?" I asked, gradually elevating my tone.

"Best keep your wits about you, for sure." He calmly replied.

After a few minutes of enjoying the views through the chopper's open doors and windows, with the wind sweeping across my face, peering out at the turquoise ocean and unspoiled sandy beaches bordered by dense green jungle, leading up to steep cliffs hundreds of feet above the crashing waves, my guided tour resumed –

"You'll see Hue, it's a city coming up. Nearby, we have a base. It's called NSA (Naval Support Activity) in Phu Bai."

"How incredible!" I exclaimed.

Flying over all of these little fishing villages with orderly rows of thatched-roof houses set on stilts with dainty boats moored to wooden docks, I espied dozens of circular mounds in the off-white soil.

"Hey Doug, are those bomb craters down there?" I called on the intercom.

"Graves. The Vietnamese bury their dead in round graves."

Over Hue, I saw the Perfume river, then the massive palace and citadel complex. That was the headquarters of our allies – the ARVN, Army of Republic of Vietnam. That's who, along with Korean, Australian and New Zealand military forces, were our comrades in arms.

"Go when you rotate to Phu Bai," came a suggestion.

Early in the conflict, in April of 1965, the Marines had established Phu Bai as a forward operating base. At the time I arrived, forward operations had been moved again, this time to Dong Ha which was closer to the action.

As we approached my new home in the chopper, we flew by a wide mouth of a broad, winding river with dirty gray banks. Pointing his finger northward at the river, the gunner shouted, "DMZ! Bad shit."

With that comment, he re-focused, craning out of the window with a firm grasp of the twin triggers of the 50-cal machine gun, scanning the ground for muzzle flashes and puffs of smoke. "Just about any time you fly anywhere around here, best be prepared to fight or not make it home," he cautioned and not casually.

These guys joke and then become dead serious.

Knowing you could be – at any moment – just gone.

We landed safety, taking no enemy fire. Touching down, I sighed, one of many sighs of relief to come with each safe landing.

When I arrived in February 1967, there had been a lull in fighting, resulting in a reduction of flight operations. That gave the troops at the forward bases time to further re-enforce the infrastructure, including their bunkers, against enemy infantry incursions, mortar barrages and rocket or artillery attacks.

Many of the structures were partially buried and all of them were protected with sandbag walls and fortified metal roofs. On the front lines, we were regularly bombarded. They'd kill a few of us. They'd injure many others. Whatever they destroyed, we immediately re-built.

And, we'd give it right back through our own shock and awe.

When enemy fighters successfully invaded one of our bases, they tried to blow up what they could, steal what weapons and ammunition they were able to carry, and fight with us hand to hand in attempts to kill or injure as many of us as they could, without any consideration given to the probability of losing their own life.

We'd kill a bunch of them. In swarms, others continued to come. Many were just teenagers.

This was the world I was entering.

Welcome to the Armpit of Armpits

Landing in Dong Ha, like other areas I'd seen, I noticed how the landscape had been denuded of any vegetation. What was once a lush forest and thick grasslands had been sprayed with chemical defoliant. It now looked like a barren moonscape. Exiting the chopper, I grabbed my bags and headed to the dispensary. Meeting me there were Art Lochridge, a Pensacola classmate, and two corpsmen. Art looked the same as I remembered, still smiling and bubbly. "Hi Al, welcome to the armpit of armpits. It's your turn to baby-sit these asshole jarheads. I've been up here a month, and all I've seen is a few sore throats and a hangnail." The two corpsmen chuckled along with him.

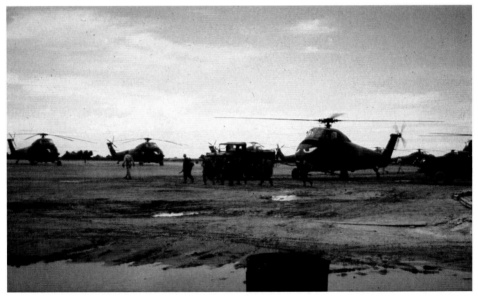

USMC Sikorsky UH-34D helicopters on the flight line in Dong Ha (Credit: Levin Archive)

"It's been quiet here, huh?" I asked.

He paused a moment and then confessed, "Yeah, but rumor has it there's a whole division of North Vietnamese Regular Army just northwest of Khe Sanh. If that's true, you guys might be in a world of hurt soon."

"Been too boring for you guys? Saved the action for me? Thanks!" I sarcastically replied.

"We aim to please, man. Anyway, I'm all packed. I'm taking the next train out. So long, sucker," he retorted with a sardonic smile. "Seriously, Al, it's been quiet and we're always hearing rumors. I wouldn't pay much attention." Two guys walked up as Art continued, "Your corpsmen, Miller and Langotti, are great guys. They'll get you situated." They immediately extended their hands. I also sensed they'd have my back.

Meeting My Awesome Corpsmen

"Hi Doc, I'm Frank Miller and this here's Jim Langotti. We'll get you squared away. Don't sweat the Lieutenant here – he likes to bullshit," Frank winked. "I got some work to do here, so Jim will show you around the base. When you guys get back, I'll clue you in on the real action here."

Frank was a big hulk of a man, about thirty-five – much older than the others and yet only a Petty Officer Second Class. Obviously, in his Navy career, he'd been busted a few times. He stood six foot two with a large paunchy belly, which was so unusual in Vietnam, where everyone was lean. His flushed face displayed a red bulbous nose, indicative of heavy alcohol ingestion. His whole demeanor bespoke a happy drunk, a warm, friendly and helpful person.

"Come on, Doc, I'll give you a tour of the base," Jim Langotti offered as he opened the screen door and gestured for me to follow.

"Thanks Art. See you in a month," I said as I started to follow the corpsman out of the dispensary.

U.S. Marines - On the Cheap

"Just a minute, Al." Art had turned serious. "I've got to clue you in on a few things before I leave you here alone. These Marines are out of their minds. They pride themselves on being able to fight a war on the cheap. Their medical budget is razor thin. That means we have to practice medicine by begging and stealing. We're always short on medical supplies and equipment here. When we go on R&R or to the Air Force and Army bases, we always 'liberate' antibiotics et cetera. It's

63

a standing joke. The Docs look at us like their poor cousins. That's ridiculous because the Marines need more medical care than any other fighting force around.

We even do better getting supplies from the black market than from our regular supply chains. There's also the NSA hospital at Danang. It's Navy, so they're well supplied. Don't ask for anything sophisticated like whole blood. We can't use it here. We have no sterility, no anesthesia, no clean water, no reliable refrigeration, and no real medicines. All we have are IV fluids for temporary blood loss replacement."

In his book, *Marine Helo*, David M. Petteys, a Vietnam helicopter pilot who was awarded the Distinguished Flying Cross and who flew with the HMM 265 in Vietnam, writes "The entire leadership here has expressed acute inability to foresee and plan for coming needs. The attitude seems to be 'take it a day at a time and play it by ear.' It's interesting the Colonels don't have any problems organizing Officer's Clubs and obtaining whiskey and ice machines." Among the rank and file, we saw where the money flowed, and where it didn't.

Dirt Floors and Sandbag Walls

While running Medevac helicopter missions, we also operated bunkered field hospitals with dirt floors, sandbag walls and a tin roof. We differentiated between triage and surgery by the number of flyswatters on the wall. Equipment and supplies were barely what we required and we had to improvise at times. Because these field hospitals were located in areas of combat activity, in the operating rooms we also kept helmets, flak jackets, and rifles at the ready. Sterility was nearly impossible with iodine being our only solution.

When a critically wounded man was rushed to these facilities, the surgical procedures consisted mostly of keeping a man breathing with a tracheostomy and oxygen, stopping major arterial bleeding, amputations, crude debridements – cutting away dead tissue and attempting to clean foreign matter out of the wounds – and applying pressure bandages. More advanced care was available in Danang at the Naval Support Activity Hospital or the USS Repose, our offshore medical hospital ship.

On the battlefield, focus is placed on physical survival. Little attention can be or is paid to the psychological trauma of combat action. In the *Navy Medicine in Vietnam* publication, by Jane K. Herman at the Naval History and Heritage Command, Lt. William Mahaffey, a Charlie Med anesthesiologist reflected that:

"Not all causalities could be repaired with scalpels and sutures. As in all wars, the stress of combat, with all its horrific by-products – took a toll on the human psyche. In Vietnam, men broke down, became contentious or grew increasingly depressed. Units sometimes spent weeks in the bush living, fighting and enduring an inhospitable environment. These surroundings took the form of heat, humidity, insects, snakes, leaches, booby traps and an invisible but deadly enemy. For the men defending isolate hilltops and outposts, enemy shelling deprived men of sleep, leaving them exhausted, disoriented and unable to function. Everyday confrontation with fear, violence, trauma, the loss of friends and their mortality sometimes left even the best fighters worn out and burned out."

As for the medical caregivers, due to collapse or indifference, was there an occasion where a Marine was lost? Surely so, at times. That would be expected.

Mahaffey was asked, "Did anyone fall between the cracks?" His direct answer was, "No. We took care of everybody."

We Ain't Got Water While the Fat Cats Get Rich

Looking at our medical facilities, you'd wonder how did we ever perform at the level we did? Simple enough. We are U.S. Marines. We do whatever it takes with whatever we have. Loyalty. Duty. Sacrifice.

During my initial base tour, listening to Art's comments, I'd chuckle when I thought he had to be kidding me, then his tone intensified. "No shit, Al, I'm serious. These Marines are so fucking cheap that when we moved into Phu Bai a couple of months ago, we didn't even have a water well – no source of fresh water at all! We drained the Army's swimming pool for drinking water. Here we are at the DMZ, you're the only doctor in the squadron, and you have no vehicle. We have one ambulance for emergencies that you have to requisition, in triplicate, *for emergencies.*

That's no problem, though, because it never runs. What you have to do is steal the Operations Officer's jeep when you need wheels in a hurry. It's okay – he told me to do it. It burns me up the way tons of money get poured into the Army and Air Force. They have fixed facilities put up by that fucking construction company where Lady Bird owns a stake. What's the name?" He looked up at Frank, who had returned to catch the closing to his tirade against greed and corruption in the U.S. military industrial complex.

"Either Brown and Root or RMK-BRJ," Frank answered.

"Or both. Anyhow, we have to live in squalor and fly shitty helicopters because the Marines don't have enough political clout."

"Wait a minute, man, what's this about Lady Bird?" I asked.

"Hey, Al, what were you doing all those months in the real world? Why do you think it's dragged on so long? Everybody here says it's the only war we have, so make it last. Big bucks to be made here, my friend. That wouldn't be so bad if we'd get ours. The Army flies Hueys where the combat's cooled down, and our Medevac guys have to take those old flying rattletraps into hot zones all the time. You'll see. This place will drive you crazy." Though smiling, Art looked disgusted. "Good luck, and keep your shit together, man."

Taking a Walk Around Base

After Art's highly irreverent version of a benediction, we exchanged a firm handshake. I went out the door to follow the corpsman Jim Langotti, a tall, skinny kid with a face covered with pimples, a residuum of moderately severe teenage acne. With a long, hooked nose and big brown eyes, the gangly kid looked as though he'd been caught up in the war frenzy right after his high school graduation. We started by walking east toward a series of concrete-block bunkers.

"In the olden days, Dong Ha used to be just a peaceful little fishing village," he told me as he led me on his version of a base tour. "This whole area used to be real dense rain forest. Must have been a beautiful place.

When the French invaded around a hundred years ago, this place became an army fortress. When the Japs took over, they used it as a military outpost, too. When Uncle Ho kicked their ass out, this was considered the northern-most military post in South Vietnam. The river's the DMZ. We're going to the old French bunker system over there. We use it as an ammo dump. You can see all the shells stacked up there."

We came upon a large, walled compound, octagonal in shape with eight-foot-high stone fencing. Wide openings on each of the eight sides contained remnants of old wooden gates that had long since rotted away. In the center stood a bunker with slit windows for rifles. Piles of artillery and mortar shells, together with rockets for the helicopter gunships, stood in the expansive yard surrounded by the fortified perimeter. Marine sentries manned two-gun towers. "They keep the big stuff in the center bunker, the little stuff out here in the yard. The gooks would love to hit this dump, but so far they haven't been able to get close enough. You see those tents and tanks back there? That's field headquarters for the Third Marine Division. That keeps 'em out."

He added, "Now I'll show you your hootch."

We turned around and headed for several wooden buildings. "Frank and I dug you a bunker cause you'll surely need it," he said with self-congratulation in his demeanor. His comment set me aback as he'd dropped it like a hospitable host would tell a guest he'd just hung clean towels in the bathroom.

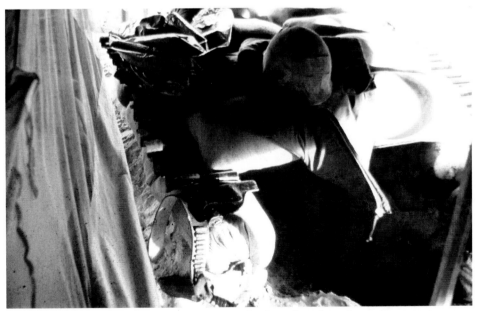

Lt. Levin's fortified bunker located adjacent to his hootch and cot for ready access in case of enemy attack with helmet, gun and flak jacket within easy reach (Credit: Levin Archive)

We Dug It for You

"Holy shit, what do you mean, a 'bunker?'"

Pointing to it, Jim responded, obviously quite proud of his generous hospitality. "A bunker, you know. When it starts raining mortar rounds or artillery shells, it'll save your ass. You see, it's personal size – a three by six hole in the ground about three feet deep with a couple of rows of sandbags around the top. It's right by your bunk so you can roll right in, if you need to, and you will need to in a hurry. It ain't like Marble or Phu Bai, where you have to run to the one closest to you, like a scared-ass motherfucker. It's right here."

We stepped by the bunker and into the hootch, which was just big enough to hold four canvas cots, two on each end, with wooden walls just up to the base of the cots with the rest wide-open window covered with canvas curtains. It was easy to see how you could just roll off the cot and fall over the wall and into the bunker in one fluid motion.

Jim grinned knowingly as he instructed, "You keep your guns, helmet, and flak jacket handy. If the scuttlebutt comes down that there'll be any action, you sleep with your fatigues and boots on. It's easy, Doc. You'll get the hang of it."

"I thought everyone said it's been quiet up here!" I nervously re-iterated.

"It has, so far. Frank and me, we got our experience at Con Thien and Gio Linh – they're two firebases near here. Activity's been going on around there for a couple months. Word has it that the RA (North Vietnamese Regular Army) is getting involved in the action. They're a lot different from the Cong locals. The Cong wear those black pajamas and straw hats. The RA wear green fatigues and helmets. The Cong hit and run. The RA hit and keep on hitting. If they're in it, we've got to be ready, so we've all been preparing for the worst-case scenario. Chances are, Doc, this could be just another rumor. We've been hearing rumors around here for months. Don't take it too seriously."

His voice trailed off to a barely audible mumble – "Just be ready. Doc, just be ready." Those last words pierced my gut like a knife and wrung out my mind like a wet dishrag.

He kept repeating 'Just be ready. Just be ready.'
Then I realized —

Shit, he's scared, too.

Wrapping up the conversation, Jim continued with a distinct resignation, "Anyway, this is where you'll stay. We'll go back to the dispensary now, and I'll bring your bags here while Frank tells you about the Medevac operations."

From jovial hospitality to grave caution.

Actually, now I'm fucking terrified.

Flying to the Rescue and Leaving No Man Behind

We walked in silence towards the dispensary hootch. As we approached it, Frank came out and motioned for me to follow him. For me, every time one of these guys opened his mouth, the situation here became more ominous. But, it seemed I was about to hear just how whacko it could get.

"You know, Doc, these Marines are a little crazy. First of all, they use the Medevac mission as a morale booster. They'll risk two officers, three enlisted men, and at least one helicopter just to pick up a single wounded guy in the field. The Army won't let their choppers in unless the combat cools down. Sometimes we go in under fire. It's crazy, but they say it makes the grunts feel better. It keeps morale up to have the Medevac choppers right there with them in battle. Just imagine big

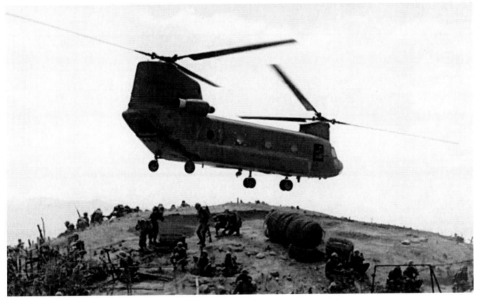

CH-47 arriving at landing zone with awaiting USMC troops (Credit: USMC)

ugly me, a morale booster. What a crock! Come on, let's go over to the flight line where I can show you the birds."

In the U.S. Marines, Medevac operations are based on the tradition of leave no man behind. It's true that no one thought twice about it. Whatever it took. Even if it meant, when short a corpsman, that doctors would go into battle. Everyone on front line considered themselves expendable.

As Marines, we were always stretched thin. That was certainly our situation. We went with what we had. And, yes, grunts knew we'd be coming if they needed us. It does boost morale. But, it also saved lives. In the evolution of war, we were now able rescue a wounded soldier in active combat and evacuate him to a medical hospital in a matter of minutes.

Routine, Priority and Emergency

Our Medevac missions were classified into three types. A Routine Medevac was just that, moving a wounded soldier from one quiet area to another for special medical treatment. This mission could be performed by any helicopter and was often done by the higher-ranking officers who, of course, flew the nicer birds. The Priority Medevac involved a man badly wounded in combat who needed to be evacuated but could survive until the landing zone was free of active combat for at least one hour. The Priority was riskier than the Routine Medevac because, although an area had quieted down, the enemy often was hiding, waiting to ambush our chopper when we arrived. Finally, the Emergency Medevac was called when the wounded grunt could not survive the hour-long wait. The area was active and everyone knew the chopper would be fired upon coming into and out of the zone.

As Frank carefully explained to me –

"The worst part is the gooks know when they've wounded our guys, that we'll call for choppers. The birds are so predictable. The gooks know we have to land and climb out into the wind, so they just get upwind of the LZ and wait for us to pull out. Then, just when we're most vulnerable, climbing low and slow, they open fire on us."

Ass Insurance

After such an ominous report, the "gift" Frank then proffered, discomforted me as much as had Langotti's news that they'd dug me my own bomb shelter to help prevent me from getting blown to pieces.

"I'm gonna give you some ass insurance," Frank smiled broadly. 'This is a sixteen-inch square piece of half-inch thick armor plate to sit on while aboard the chopper. It's pretty heavy to carry around, but you'll be glad you've got it. When the gooks fire up at you, the rounds can come through the belly. A 50 cal will blow you out of the chopper. Nothing can stop that. But ass insurance will stop a 30 cal from coming up your butt. You know nobody survives that kind of hit, which blows shit all through your belly and pulverizes your pancreas. Out here, nobody lives through that. Nobody."

Roger that, Frank.

After what you just described, I won't leave home without it!

Our Marine Corps Choppers

During my tour of duty, we were utilizing three types of helicopters – the oldest was the creaky UH-34D, a Sikorsky helicopter, in service for ten years. Although it had probably been a good bird in its time, it had limited load-carrying capabilities, being powered by a single piston engine. It carried the optimal crew of four: pilot, co-pilot, crew chief and door gunner. The guns were 7.62mm M-60 machine guns, one fixed to the front window on the left side and the other mounted to the forward bulkhead of a large door on the right side – primarily used as defensive weapons only marginally effective in laying down a barrage of fire to keep the enemy's head down while the bird was maneuvering into and out of landing zones.

This chopper had a large, four-bladed single main rotor that made a loud WHOOSHing noise when it cut through the air. Anybody could tell it was coming for miles in quiet jungles. Because these birds were abundant and inexpensive, the Marine Corps utilized them extensively on Medevac missions, where they would carry a medical corpsman as special crew to minister to the wounded while the gunner and crew chief protected the aircraft during an enemy onslaught. On cold days, the bird could generate enough lift to evacuate as many

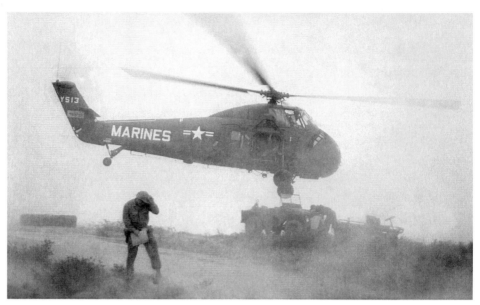
UH-34D landing in a dust cloud, delivering supplies to front line soldiers (Credit: USMC)

as four wounded men. On hot ones it could sometimes hardly handle a single soldier.

As Frank described it –

"When it's hot, the old bird shudders and shakes, almost popping a hemorrhoid coming out of a landing zone."

Shuddering Shithouses and Flying Flash Bulbs

Frank also introduced me to the two nicknames these birds had earned. Because they'd vibrate tremendously as they lumbered into the air, even chattering your teeth, while reeking strongly of hydraulic fluid and gasoline, the guys generally called them "shuddering shit-houses." Their other nickname proved more chillingly ironic. Frank pointed to the skin of the chopper – "Parts of this here skin are made of magnesium, to save weight, the same stuff they put in flash bulbs. This bird will blow up in flames when an incendiary round hits the hull. We call it the 'flying flash bulb.'"

"Are you kidding? Why would the military let us fly planes into combat that blow up with incendiary rounds?" I asked.

He looked at me startled, unbelieving, as if I'd let him down. I suddenly realized I'd asked a stupid question. He finally deigned to answer.

"Doc, you should know better by now. You don't get to be a General or an Admiral by knowing about combat. You get there by kissing ass. The right ass at the right time. Why now, in fucking Dong Ha, do I have to tell you all this shit? Why didn't any of us get told this in the Stateside training?" he asked angrily. "I'll tell you why. The guys that kissed ass best, got to stay in the States to train us asshole losers. They don't know combat from Shinola. Forget the clueless training command. Listen to me and you might stay alive."

We walked around to the door of the chopper and Frank nodded toward the inside. "You see this forward bulkhead there?" he asked, pointing to the forward wall of the crew compartment.

"Ahead and below is the engine. A round that hits us usually gets hung up there before it penetrates the crew compartment. Going in and coming out of zones, forget about anything or anyone else. Just sit there on your ass insurance with your back to that bulkhead. That way you're covered from the front and the bottom. I've never seen rounds come through the back of the chopper. So, the only place you're really vulnerable to taking a round is from the sides, and you can usually survive a small arms hit from there."

"Come on, I'll show you the better birds now."

We walked down the airstrip towards a much bigger helicopter that looked like a well-designed flying banana. It had two massive three-bladed rotors, one fore and one aft. Doors in the front were for the pilot and co-pilot. It had a large aft ramp for loading the crew and payloads.

I was really impressed with its sleek and modern design.

What a Bird!

The CH-46A was new, a Boeing-built twin jet turbine-powered helicopter. In late 1966, it was first introduced into combat. The aircraft's giant rotors provided a great deal of lift. They also produced a roaring WHOPPing sound. Its crew was manned by a pilot and co-pilot plus a crew chief and gunner, who operated the two door-mounted 50 caliber machine guns. Frank walked over to one of the machine guns mounted in the forward window on the left side. "These are real offensive weapons." Picking up a bandolier of 50 caliber rounds, he

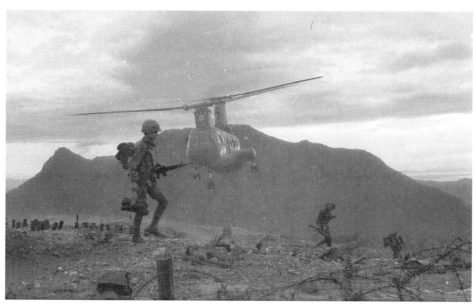

Boeing CH-46 delivers troops on patrol (Credit: USMC)

pointed to the various swatches of paint on each of the rounds.

"These colors mark the different kind of bullets. Blue is armor-piercing balls, white is Willy Peter – white phosphorus incendiary rounds – red is explosive, and black is fragmenting antipersonnel rounds. The bandoliers have one red, one white, and one blue, with two blacks in each five rounds. The Willy Peters are the tracers. These mothers do some major damage. You can really tear up what's below you with these things. You hit a guy in the midsection with an explosive round and you blow him in two pieces. They use these birds for hot troop inserts. They can carry up to sixteen grunts with full combat loads of gear and ammo. Sometimes we get them for Medevacs when the 34's are busy. A word of warning, though. Look at this." He pointed down at the chopper's sturdy looking waffle-grated floor. "This looks good, but it won't stop a butter knife. We call it morale plate. So, don't forget your ass insurance."

Huey's Hellish Firestorm

Bringing the real firepower, the third Marine helicopter used in combat at that time was the UH-1E, affectionately known as the "Huey" – "one mean machine," Frank assured me. Twin turbojet engines powered these magnificent birds built by Bell, with a large

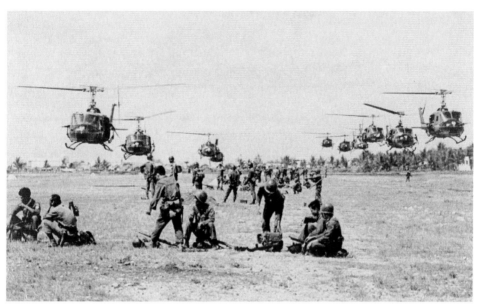

Group of UH-1 Hueys transporting ground troops (Credit: U.S. Army)

twin-bladed main rotor that slapped through the air with a characteristic, unmistakable and loud WHOP-WHOP-WHOP sound. Hueys were powerful and amazingly maneuverable.

Although the Army used them extensively for Medevac missions, the Marine Corps didn't have enough Hueys to go around, so the Marines utilized them mainly as gunships. They were equipped with two door-mounted M-60 machine guns and two skid-mounted rocket pods containing six projectiles each. This lethal aircraft also had two nose-mounted 7mm rapid fire machine guns operated by the pilot and co-pilot. It carried a hell of a lot of ammo and could lay down a carpet of fire about as wide as a football field. We used them as vital ground support aircraft for troop operations and as gun support to protect the Medevac missions.

Frank stroked the nose of the bird tenderly.

"These Hueys are always the first up in the air on the Medevac alert. You'll hear two Hueys orbiting over our ready room hootch before you hear anybody holler 'Medevac.' The squadron gets the first call and decides whether to go or not go. The WHOP-WHOP of this motherfucker is one sound you'll never forget. It wakes you up no matter how sound you're asleep. It means Medevac. They'll be airborne while we load into our 34, or, if we're lucky, a 46."

Launching a Medevac Mission

When the decision to launch a Medevac mission was made, the pilot got the briefing while the co-pilot ran like hell out to the bird and started its engines. The crew boarded the chopper with the co-pilot. Since everything was ready, these birds were up and running in seconds. Two Hueys would orbit our landing pad while we loaded into our UH-34D or occasionally our CH-46A to fly off on the mission. Another helicopter always accompanied the Medevac chopper – it acted as the chase plane. The Medevac mission flight, therefore, consisted of four aircraft: the Medevac helicopter, the chase plane (usually another bird of the same type), and two Huey gunships.

When the flight reached the LZ, the gunships would orbit at an altitude of about five hundred feet. These helicopters would carefully survey the area for enemy activity. The Medevac bird, with its corpsman aboard, would then drop into the zone while the chase plane orbited at an altitude of two hundred feet. If the Medevac bird got hit and went down, as it often did, the Hueys would lay down a ring of fire to keep the gooks busy while the chase plane swooped in to rescue the crew of the stricken bird.

"Frank, how many Medevacs have you flown?" I asked.

"About thirty so far," he responded.

"How many times have you taken fire?"

"About a dozen."

"How many medevacs has Art, Dr. Lochridge, flown so far?"

"About a dozen."

"How many times has he taken fire?" I asked.

He responded hesitantly –

"Well, there were a couple of bad ones. His bird went down once and exploded. They lost the gunner, but the rest of them made it back."

Why Send a Doctor on a Medevac Flight?

"No wonder he's so bitter," I interjected. "How come a doctor has to fly a Medevac?"

"I was up on a Medevac when Eddie Lang, one of our corpsmen, got killed north of Gio Linh last month. They called an emergency, and the Doc had to go. But we've got Langotti now as a replacement."

"What do you mean he *had* to go?", I asked as I was thinking that normally flight surgeons don't go out on Medevac flights. That is the job of the corpsmen.

"Lieutenant," Frank looked at me with soulful eyes, "with all due respect to your education and your rank, they mean nothing to the Marines. As far as they're concerned, when they need you, you're just another grunt."

"You mean they'll order me to go on a mission?" I asked.

"Doc, I've been up here for five months now and I ain't heard nobody order nobody around. Up here rank means squat. We've got a job to do and we're all watching out for each other. These guys are like my brothers. I can't let them down. Doc Lochridge feels that way too. That's why he's so pissed. He don't like seeing his brothers wasted."

Then, Frank peered into my eyes directly and intently.

"Nobody forces you. You just go because that's what they expect. I wouldn't do this shit, but these are good guys and nobody in the real world gives a damn about them. They're sending us out here with crap so they can make big money in the States. These guys need me and I'm gonna help them. If my big ugly face raises their morale, then that's that. You handle this your way, Doc. Nobody'll force you to do nothing."

I stood there quietly.

What will I do?

How the hell am I going to survive?

I won't.

Still in disbelief that this atrocity had been thrust upon me, acceptance and then anger would be rapidly approaching. As Frank and I entered the base's living area, he pointed towards my hootch where Langotti had loaded my bags on a cot. I shook Frank's hand. He looked me squarely in the eye and squeezed tightly –

"You'll see what I mean Doc. You will know what to do. You may hate the candyasses above us, but you'll like these guys."

Frank was right. I did. They were and continue to be my inspiration – the Marine Corps Medevac crews and corpsmen who put their lives on the line for their comrades, to treat the wounded and to save lives.

When the call came and they needed me, I never hesitated.

Chapter Five
Medevacs: Practicing Medicine While Fighting

"Do No Harm. Do Know Harm."
USMC Corpsman Motto

By late that afternoon, I'd managed to organize my hootch. I wandered out to the flight line to see if I could meet some of the pilots who happened to be around. As I entered the ready room shack, I encountered two of them straddling a long bench facing each other. Between them sat a makeshift backgammon board over which they appeared locked in an intense championship game.

Watching the action, Doug McAllister noticed my arrival and bolted upright, offering me his best John Wayne salute and hollering, "Geeentlemen – and I use that term veeery loosely – I would like to introduce our new flight quack, Lieeuteenent Levin of the UUUnited States Naavy." All of the pilots immediately stood at stiff attention, folded up their arms with their hands in their armpits to mimic bird wings and started quacking. Then the whole room turned into a momentary aviary with grown men jumping around, flapping their "wings," and quacking like maniacal ducks.

Art Lochridge was right, these guys were crazy.

After the startling explosion of their total zaniness subsided, the guys good-naturedly began introducing themselves. Lieutenant Larry Kozar was a little Jewish kid from the Bronx, the only Jewish guy on the base, so when he found a *Lantzman* – a countryman – he immediately warmed up with wise cracks. "Hey Doc, how good are you at plastic surgery? Lochridge tried to make the Heap here beautiful, but he fucked up. Can you help?" He pointed to big Bob Boisheid, an enormous guy who'd played first string left tackle for the University of Texas before he joined the Marines. Nicknamed "The Heap" in flight school, although he rose to the rank of captain and plane commander, he still good-naturedly carried the moniker and took the ribbing.

Feeling compelled to respond, I offered, "I'm lousy on plastic surgery, but my specialty is circumcisions. I did a lot at Pensacola and Camp Pendleton. Every Marine that pisses into his left hip pocket had a Levin clip job, until proven otherwise." That got things warmed up, and we'd become fast buddies by the time for chow. The mess hall was not as nice as that at Marble, but even up here the food still proved quite acceptable. However, no O Club. Not in combat areas, where a sober soldier is a fighting soldier.

After dinner, Barney Whalen, a big Irishman, came over to our table and sat down next to us, looking worried, but Larry nevertheless brightly started up –

"Barney, I'd like you to meet the new healer from the East. Our new quack makes two Jew boys in the squadron. Better watch out, pretty soon we're gonna outnumber you Guinea wops."

"You asshole, can't you kikes tell the difference between an Australian and an Irishman?" he guffawed.

"I don't know, with your pants down you all look the same," Larry retorted.

After a chuckle between us, Barney changed to a serious tone.

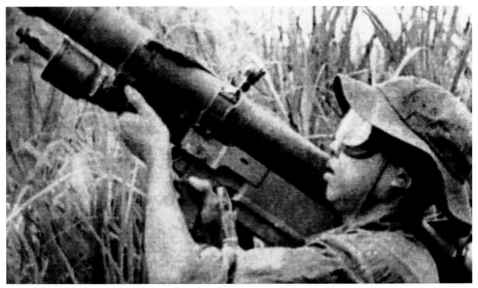

NVA soldier takes aim with a Soviet-made NVA shoulder fired missile (Source: USAF)

"You guys better know – Operations says the NVA's infiltrating. They're north of Khe Sanh."

Noting that North Vietnamese Regular Army was far more formidable than the Viet Cong, he warned of an impending enemy blitzkrieg.

"We've got patrols engaging enemies wearing NVA green uniforms. Regular army. Well-armed and trained. Not just Viet Cong. We're beefing up the border guards. You guys better sleep with your boots on."

Though we all slept in our flight suits and combat boots, that night proved quiet, permitting some peaceful-enough shut eye. I could've never anticipated the extreme level of physical and mental exhaustion I would soon experience.

Medevac Flight Planning

Around 5:30 the next morning I woke up, headed down to the small shower hootch for my morning cleanup and then to breakfast. Since the dispensary had no regular hours at Dong Ha, I decided to wander to the flight line to kibbitz with the pilots. On that clear morning the ready room shack buzzed with activity. The pilots got briefed on various missions, chose call signs, and plotted their courses. It amazed me to see how well these guys knew the terrain. Instead of using radials and compass headings, they talked about ridges and hills and river bends. The plane commanders up here had flown enough in-country to become intimately familiar with the area. This was vital because reliable radio navigation aids in the I Corps were nearly non-existent.

WHOP-WHOP-WHOP

Then I heard it – the distinctive sound of the Huey gunships orbiting over the ready room hootch. Then the cry, "Medevac! Medevac!" as a corporal from the communications shack two hootches down burst through the door and ran into the room thrusting a sheet of paper at Major John Schneider, the operations officer.

"Who's up for this one?" Schneider shouted.

Jumping into action, a young-looking captain in the corner of the room, Jack House, ran up to Schneider while his co-pilot Marty

Methuen sprinted out the door to start up their aircraft's engines. I caught a glimpse of the crew chief, the gunner, and Frank Miller, the corpsman, racing towards the chopper, now coming angrily to life.

I moved closer to continue listening to the briefing. I was able to see the message that arrived. It was typed in one-line code with capital letters and numbers. "Today's code is Delta, so the coordinates are India November Echo and Alpha Alpha Charlie. This is a class two priority NSA. The smoke is Foxtrot," Schneider said.

Then, he pulled out a whiz wheel, the wheel-shaped decoder, and turned the outside wheel until the letter D came into the window. He then looked down the long slit in the wheel and read off the numbers that showed up in the space adjacent to the letters on the message. These were the numbers of the map coordinates, which Jack copied onto the paper of his knee board – the small clip board the pilots strapped to their legs for writing while in flight.

Then they both turned to the wall map hanging behind the desk. Dong Ha was marked with a compass rose that had a nail in its center from which hung a long cord marked with blue ink lines, in scale, of kilometers. Jack found the location of the coordinates on the map that marked the LZ – the landing zone he had to reach. Then he extended the cord taut to that point and counted the number of marks from the center nail to his finger and said, "I get 27 clicks (kilometers) on the 235 radial of Dong Ha."

Schneider called out, "Foxtrot is three, and that's yellow. You're Sky Shadow one and two, and the guns are Hijack one and two. The chase and gun ships will split on your signal." Jack nodded his head and bolted out of the door in a dead run to the chopper now ready to launch. The briefing had taken less than a minute. The entire Medevac got airborne and in route in less than three minutes.

Coding Our Mission Communications

"What kind of a run is that?" I asked Schneider.

Showing me the coded communication, he explained:

"This is our code. The enemy monitors our radio communications, so every day we get two sets of numbers broadcast to the units in the field. These match up with a list of numbers hand-delivered to the field commanders in sealed envelopes every week. We open an envelope for each day. And if we open any envelope prematurely, special couriers bring a new set. The first broadcast number lines up with the number in the envelope. That number tells which letter to put under the top window of the whiz wheel to find the map coordinates. You see, we broadcast the number twenty-seven today. In today's envelope twenty-seven lines up with the number five."

On another sheet of paper, there were two columns of numbers. He pointed to the number twenty-seven, adjacent to which appeared the number five. "This means the fifth letter is the one we put under the top of the whiz wheel. All of the rest of the first seven letters correspond to the letters along the side of this slit in the wheel." He pointed to its long slit. "You can see as I turn the wheel, the numbers next to the letters change. The seventh letter is F, or Foxtrot. Here, F is next to the number three. This week, three means yellow smoke."

He then pointed to a list of colors with numbers next to them. "That tells you what color smoke the ground troops will pop. They have a bunch of colored smoke grenades: yellow, white, red, green, and blue. When they hear the Medevac flight coming, they pop the designated color smoke grenade, which lets the pilots know exactly where the LZ is.

Once in a while, the enemy breaks the code and you see five yellow smokes popped at the same time. That's when the pilots get creative. They ask sports questions like, 'Give me the Packers.' The gooks don't know the Packers are from Green Bay, so the green smoke is ours. If the ground calls, 'You got it,' and there's only one green smoke, you're okay. If not, we try something else.

The second broadcast number is the code for the Medevac patients. Today's number is one. That means that one is emergency, two is priority and three is routine. This is an emergency Medevac taking one guy to NSA in Danang. He probably needs surgery urgently. I gave Jack the call signs for himself and the chase plane and the call signs for the gun ships. Since they'll be going into NSA in a secure zone, the Hueys and the chase plane will split off and return when Jack signals that he's safely airborne. They'll come back here because things seem to be heating up out there."

"They're All Dead"

Within thirty minutes I heard the sound of choppers again and the cry come out.

"Medevac! Medevac!"

This time, something was different. I was uncertain why, but I could sense it. Normally they circled while awaiting the Medevac chopper to take off. This time the Huey gunships landed in front of the ready room hootch and while the rotors turned at idle, the pilots of both ships ran in. Our Medevac pilots and the Huey pilots confabbed with Schneider and reviewed the map pointing to a location just below the DMZ, about twenty miles to the west of our position. While they conferred, I saw Jim Langotti and the Medevac crew running towards their chopper.

After the conference, which took no more than five minutes, all of the pilots ran for their birds, and the flight was off, already with a full crew. I was not needed. As they departed, I heard Major Schneider call out –

"This is an emergency job. Four grunts tripped a Bouncing Betty. Those damn 151mm artillery shells, rigged as land mines. When the wire's tripped, the shell shoots up and blows around waist high. These guys caught it real bad, but there was no fire fight in the area. I hope the gooks stay gone so we get in and out with no trouble."

"Wow!" I exclaimed, trying to figure out what I'd do in a mess like that, realizing that I really didn't have a clue.

But, my wake-up call to action came soon enough.

In the ready room, Schneider and I were trying to relax, playing a game of acey deucey, a simple betting card game. But just after we started, the corporal from the communications shack came through the door, this time walking, not running. "Major, they got that last bird with small arms. It went down with a lot of battle damage. The grunts surrounded it and all aboard survived. Everyone but the crew chief is coming back on the chase plane. He's staying with the chopper to repair it. We should be ready to dispatch parts as soon as we get an assessment of the battle damage."

"What about the wounded?" I asked.

"They're all dead. They died before the chopper got there. The bird that delivers the spare parts to them should bring back the KIAs." Perhaps as some protection from the cruelties of reality, that acronym for "killed in action" always replaced anything simpler like or "corpses" or "deceased."

"Okay, thanks Corporal," Schneider responded with a shaky voice. "We'll have to wait for the call on the damage before we can take any action."

I got up from the bench and walked to the door of the ready room hootch. My first full day there and I was completely unnerved as I begin to fully realize what is ahead.

It's really bad.

Time seemed to drag. Where was Miller? Why didn't Langotti make it back? Would they in fact return?

Doc, Are You Ready?

Fear washed over me like a tidal wave. My gut was wrenching. Then the word came – Jim Langotti, that tall, skinny kid who hadn't yet outgrown his pimples, had taken a round in his left testicle, while on the aft ramp loading stretchers. He was okay, and was now in route to the Charlie Med for treatment.

Frank Miller, where the hell are you? I screamed silently to myself.

Then, that now familiar roar – *WHOP-WHOP-WHOP.* "Medevac! Medevac! Emergency!" Bursting into the shack, the corporal handed the paper to Schneider, who studied it briefly, while Bob Bolsheid and Marty Lang jumped into action. He looked at me and asked, "Doc, can you make this one?"

"Yeah, if nobody minds a rank novice aboard," I responded. Then, I hesitated, "Wait a minute, I don't have my equipment."

"Here's a Unit 1," Jerry Kemp inserted. He was one of the pilots in the hootch who threw the bag of medical supplies at me. "Take my helmet and cement shirt," he added.

"Thanks, man!" I shouted, bolting out of the door towards the waiting chopper. As I ran and tried to collect my wits, I commenced a dialogue with myself.

What the hell am I doing?
I can get killed doing this!

Why?

Stop, Levin!

Levin!

My body was running and my mind was racing, but they were out of sync. I began to feel schizoid – one part of me a mindless automaton that responded to gut-level instincts and the other a rational human that was terrified for his own life.

Which person would dominate?

By then I had gotten to the chopper, from which crew chief Robert (Stubby) Stubblefield leaned out and shouted, "Doc, where's your gun?"

"Gun? Whaddaya mean, gun? I'm a doctor. I'm a noncombatant."

"Doc!" He yelled quite exasperated. "This is an emergency Medevac. Go and get your goddamn gun."

"Okay, but I'll have to run to my hootch to get them."

'That's okay, Doc. Here comes Miller. He can fly with us."

Then I turned around just in time to see Frank at full speed, huffing and puffing, running towards the chopper. "Doc, I'll take this one. You got the next one," he said breathlessly with a weak smile. I stood there, feeling like a horse's ass while the crew clambered aboard. Frank leaned out the door and threw me a big khaki bag with IV fluid bottles taped to the shoulder strap.

"Here," he shouted, "Take this extra Unit 1. It's loaded. You may need it. So long, see you later."

He waved a loose and silly salute as the helicopters lifted off the tarmac.

I didn't hesitate. I grabbed the Unit 1 and ran to my hootch, where I changed from combat fatigues to flight suit, grabbed my ass insurance, strapped on the .38 revolver and pulled the M-14 over my shoulder. I then snatched up my flight bag and cement shirt, broke into a dead run back to the ready room hootch. All that equipment must have weighed a good thirty pounds, but I was so pumped up. I was unfazed. I was actually quite amazed at how fast I was moving, even with my heavy load.

When I finally got to the ready room hootch again, all was quiet as I sat down to catch my breath. I was prepared for next time.

Inside a Unit 1 Medical Bag

With some spare moments, I began to look through the Unit 1 bag, which is what corpsmen carry into the battlefield. Designed for medical equipment, it had a single shoulder strap and closed with a large flap. Inside, numerous small compartments hold battle dressings, airways, and minor surgery equipment. One small compartment contained syringes and IM meds – intramuscular medications: epinephrine for shock, Benadryl for bad allergic reactions, and four vials of morphine sulfate – obviously for guys in severe pain like burns and open compound fractures.

Battle dressings of various sizes filled the main bulk of the bag – everything from abdominal pads (ABDs) to four by fours – all Marine green because white dressings made great targets at night, and the enemy would shoot at our wounded. The bag also contained a number of splints of different sizes and large rolls of adhesive tape, with the khaki canvas airway pack and the minor surgery pack at the back of the bag along with a flashlight and a mirror. These last two items were primarily used to tell whether a man was dead by checking pupil reaction and breathing.

Taped on the shoulder strap were two 250 ml. bottles of normal saline and one 150 ml. bottle of human serum albumin. Contained in a small rectangular brown cardboard box were needles and tubing, taped to each bottle, which was then wrapped with a battle dressing and attached to the shoulder strap. I figured Frank put those there for ready access. On the bottom of the strap, I found taped a six-inch length of what looked like plastic fuel pipe. One end was sharpened.

I paused to wonder what that was for.

Medevac! Medevac! – My First Mission

Familiar with my Unit 1, and feeling ready to go, again I challenged Schneider to game of acey-deucey. About half-way into the game we heard the now already familiar – the choppers circling and the call once again –

WHOP-WHOP-WHOP — Medevac! Medevac!

Charging through the door, the corporal gave Schneider the dispatch. On this mission, Jack House was the next pilot up, so he hurried up to the desk to confer with Schneider while Marty Methuen, his co-pilot, ran out to start up their chopper. The corporal turned to me. "This one's priority, but we've really got to go fast. It's the company corpsman. He took a hit but kept on working with the other wounded guys for a good hour till he collapsed. Nobody realized how bad he was hit till he fell over. The area was too hot to call for a chopper till now."

"Damn! If he took a round an hour ago and just collapsed, by now, he could be really bad off," I called out while grabbing all of my equipment and sprinting out of the door to the waiting chopper. Going in the roomier twin-rotor UH-46 because there were at least four wounded, we took off from the pad and began climbing to altitude. The crew chief closed the bottom door of the aft ramp and left the top door open, allowing the cold wind to circulate through the chopper. I ripped off two of the bottles of IV Ringer's Lactate and hung them by metal hooks to the bulkhead stringers and attached the needles and tubes, and loosely looped them upon themselves. I was ready.

Looking out the window, as we flew inland, I had a few moments to reflect.

What the hell are we all doing here?

Why waste a doctor?

Why waste any of us?

But there was no time for further contemplation. In my heightened mental state, I rehearsed everything I would do, just in case. Ready at my fingertips were my airways for a face wound or a guy choking on his tongue, the battle dressings just in case the ones applied in the field were falling off, and IV fluids prepared to replace blood loss and prevent pressure drops.

Also, I had my weapons close at hand.

In route, Methuen radioed to the grunts announcing they had the new flight quack aboard. If anybody could save their corpsman, this quack could.

No pressure, right? I whispered to myself.

Wrong!

As the walls shook with the engines spooling down, we descended rapidly into the LZ, hitting the ground in a controlled crash. Instantly the bottom door of the aft ramp dropped to the ground and two grubby-looking grunts came running towards the ramp carrying a litter. At first, all I could see were the soles of the wounded man's combat boots.

How strange.

Both of his feet are flopped over to the left.

No muscle tone.

I haven't seen this before.

When they had placed their wounded comrade on the floor of the chopper, one of the litter bearers came up to me, tightly grabbing my arm looking right at me with tears in his eyes, shaking me, crying and shouting –

"He'll be all right, won't he Doc? He's our corpsman. He'll be all right, won't he?"

"I'll do all I can. That's a promise."

Just then, three other wounded guys crowded into the chopper through the aft ramp, all boarding under their own power. One had a splint and a battle dressing on his forearm, the other two had leg wounds. The litter bearer let go of my arm and ran back out of the chopper.

Within seconds the lower door of the aft ramp came up and we started climbing out of the zone. I looked down at the corpsman on the litter. He was covered with a khaki blanket with his head and feet sticking out. His face was ashen gray and his pupils were dilated. I pulled the flashlight out of the Unit 1 and shined it in his eyes. The pupils didn't respond. I touched his conjunctiva: no reaction. His skin was cold. I put the mirror in front of his open mouth: no breath.

Now, the peculiar position of the feet made sense: this man was dead.

Looking up, I caught the glaring eyes of the other men in the chopper. These poor Marine grunts had been watching me intently, fully expecting the doctor to save their comrade. They had banked their hopes of survival in this non-miracle worker. Their buddy was laying there and I felt impotent, totally at a loss as to how to bring this son of a bitch back to life, not wanting to accept this was a lifeless, mutilated corpse that laid before us.

What do they expect of me?

Don't they know I'm as human as they are?

Tears were welling in my eyes. I was struck by the shock of the first death of a Marine whom I saw and who was one of our medical corpsman. My gut wrenched in our shared agony. I turned and vomited heavy dry heaves.

Straighten up, stinking pile of shit.

Levin! Just do your job.

Help somebody.

Taking a deep breath, and mustering what energy I had, I moved through the back of the chopper, checking the rest of the wounded. Satisfied that they were stable, I curled up on the floor of the chopper with my back to the forward bulkhead and continued to retch and weep, in moments uncontrollably.

In the chilly draft of that noisy chopper belly, I finally gathered myself as we began our descent. The gun ships and chase plane had split off and returned to Dong Ha. We were heading to our Phu Bai medical facility. Minutes later, the crew chief tapped my shoulder. "Charlie Med," he shouted.

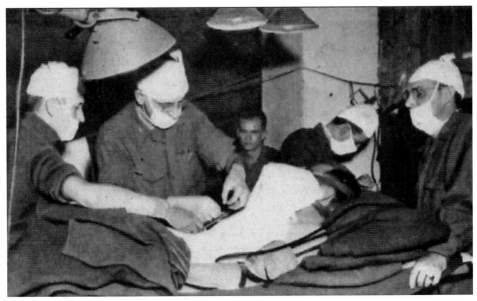

USMC flight surgeons perform surgery in Phu Bai hospital (Credit: USMC)

We landed on a large, corrugated metal helipad just outside the hospital. Four corpsmen ran toward the chopper. These guys looked like the ones Stateside, cleanly shaven, their fatigues neat and starched, with creases. Two doctors, who looked like I used to look, waited at the edge of the pad in neatly pressed fatigues with shiny silver and gold insignias on their collars. In their hands they carried stethoscopes. Nobody had helmets or flak jackets. Nobody had guns. This was the medicine that I knew. The corpsmen ran aboard the chopper – two began to help the walking wounded and two went for the litter. When I gave them the thumbs down sign over it, one nodded and they shuffled off with the KIA for processing. I leaned out the window and waved to the medical officers on the side of the pad who smiled and waved back before following the corpsmen and the walking wounded into the hospital. The crew chief tapped me on the shoulder and shouted, "We can't stop here, Doc. The captain says you can come back to visit later when it ain't so hot out there."

"I understand," I replied, as we departed for Dong Ha.

Rumors of Major Offensive Were True

Upon returning to our ready room hootch, I found that Miller was off on yet another Medevac mission. Combat activity continued to escalate. Numerous patrols reported engaging regular NVA troops in their TAOR, Tactical Area of Responsibility. Intelligence reported division-sized enemy troop movements in the A Sau Valley at the far northwest corner of Vietnam on the Laotian border.

The rumors of a massive offensive during the Tet holiday had been true. Oddly enough, everyone seemed calm and resolved. Charlie Pitman stood by himself reviewing the map on the back wall of the ready room when I approached him.

"Major," I asked, "what do you think is going to happen out there?"

"Doc, this may surprise you, but we are not unhappy about the regular army coming into this battle. You see, we've been fighting these damn Viet Cong for years. That's like trying to punch a bowl of jello. You hit and they fade back. Now that large masses of troops are involved, the battle is predictable, the enemy is identifiable. This is how we've been trained to fight. You'll see. This is where the Marines will shine. We'll kick their ass."

"Oorah," was my nervous response.

Throwing the Switch to Go Mode

WHOP-WHOP-WHOP

"Medevac, Medevac, Emergency Medevac!"

Instantaneously, your mind switches. Your body reacts. You enter the "go" mode. Execute your mission. Follow your training. Don't resist killing, when necessary. This mission, as many others, it was an emergency. No time to wait. We were heading into a hot zone. As the chopper's engines fired up, in a dead run, carrying my gear, I joined Ted Davenport, the co-pilot and crew. Jerry Kemp, the plane commander, had just gotten the briefing and was sprinting forty yards behind me.

Surely, I will die. Perhaps this is that time.

I am so scared.

I pounded my panic down. I re-gained and maintained complete focus.

Just do.

Think later.

Our crew clambered aboard and were airborne in less than three minutes. I sat on one of the canvas sling seats along the side wall of the chopper. This time I wouldn't hang up the IV bottles until I knew the Medevac was alive and needed it. Once airborne, I wondered nervously. Were these other guys like me? Were they cracking up? I felt I was on the verge.

All of a sudden, we made an abrupt course change and started a steep descent. The crew chief tapped me on the shoulder and shouted, "Hot zone, Doc, hot zone." He grabbed the handles of his 50 cal machine gun and craned out the window to scan the ground for muzzle flashes, and I grabbed my ass insurance and sat on the floor with my back against the forward bulkhead.

What a helpless feeling! All I could do was sit on that armor plating and wait for the enemy to open fire. At least, we had our machine guns.

POP-POP-POP

Responding to enemy rifle fire, the gunners opened up their 50 cals on both sides with deafening concussions and expended shells raining over me. As the entire chopper vibrated with the rattle of the guns, the distinct odor of spent gunpowder pervaded throughout the belly of the chopper, leaving a metallic taste in my mouth.

I hit the floor. Then I saw it. I saw it in slow motion. I swear to God, I saw it. A round – an enemy round – came right up through the floor. I could see it spiraling up through the cabin, no more than four feet in front of me. And behind it, like a string of spaghetti, up came a strip of the flooring that we called morale plate.

I snapped back into real time. Taking enemy hits, our chopper pulled up violently and climbed back to altitude. Our pilots elected to abort the mission and return to base to assess the aircraft's battle damage.

The Medevacs would have to wait a while longer before they could be rescued.

If they survived.

We felt like shit for not getting to them.

No Sooner We're Off Again

Just as we are arriving at Dong Ha, the gunner of another chopper crew came sprinting up to the door shouting, "Doc! Doc! Area's secured now. The grunts out there need you bad. We have another chopper waiting. Can you go out again?"

We were getting our chance to redeem ourselves.

"Sure. I'm right behind you." I grabbed my equipment and sprinted across the tarmac to the awaiting chopper. The gun ships and chase plane remained in orbit over the base until we took off for the Medevac location. I was thinking, hopefully, we wouldn't draw fire on this run. I sat back and checked my equipment. I had everything.

My mouth is dry.

Totally dry.

How long has it been since I had drink of water.

My head is pounding.

I feel sick.

My gut, something's wrong. It's rock hard.

When did I take my last dump?

Do I have paralytic ileus?

When did I shit?

How about a piss? When did I piss last?

93

Do I have renal shutdown?
Maybe I just pissed my pants?
Didn't even notice.
What's wrong?
Shit, I'm scared!
That's it, you asshole. You're terrified.
How come you volunteer for these goddamn stupid missions?
Where's your fuckin' brain?

Descending Into Utter Calamity and Chaos

Suddenly, our bird lurched to the right to begin a rapid descent to our landing zone. With the crew chief and gunner at their 50 cals, I moved quickly over onto my ass insurance with my back to the forward cabin bulkhead. We entered the zone in a typical controlled crash with the engines spooling at a fast idle. The crew chief dropped the aft ramp and immediately, in a frenzied rush, a group of grubby grunts carrying litters began to crowd aboard the chopper. They hurled four litters aboard and three walking wounded clamored inside. The last man leapt over the rising aft ramp as the engines spooled up and the chopper left the ground again. The operation was over in less than one minute.

As soon our chopper had safely climbed out of the zone, I got up to look over the guys on the litters. The first had a large ABD pad on his right abdominal flank. He looked stable but deserved an IV if I had time. The second had a chest wound over which the company corpsman had placed a plasticized occlusive patch in order to avoid problems with tension pneumothorax. In a chest wound, a flap of broken chest wall can act as a one-way valve: when the patient inhales, the valve opens and allows air to enter the chest cavity through the bullet hole. When the patient exhales, the valve closes and traps the air in the chest. Since the hole in the chest wall does not communicate with the trachea or bronchi, there is no way the air can escape, so it builds up – each breath builds more and more pressure until the chest literally explodes. This is a common problem with small arms chest wounds mostly at the missile entry site. In real-world medicine chest tubes and suction solve these problems, but that kind of treatment's impossible in the field or in a heaving chopper, so all we had were temporary tire patches. This guy needed an IV right away. The third guy looked dead, or near enough dead, that he would get my attention last, and the fourth guy had a head wound and looked unconscious. He was breathing easily and the dressing on the wound was tight enough that I didn't need to worry about him. That being the case, I pulled off the two bottles of Ringer's Lactate and easily got the IV's going on the first two guys. It was a simple task to find a vein on these muscular boys, and I let the fluids run into their veins wide open. There was no problem of fluid overload with these young men and their excellent cardiovascular systems.

Then I looked after the walking wounded. One guy had a wound through his right thigh. Although the corpsman had ripped the pant leg off and applied a large ABD pad over it, the area was beginning to swell and there was obvious deformity of the upper leg. "Did you walk on this leg?" I yelled to the man.

"Yes sir, I did." Damn it, I hated to be called sir. I wasn't a military officer. I was a doctor. Well, I couldn't let that crap bother me now.

"Didn't it hurt?"

"No sir, but it does wiggle a little."

"Wiggle! Your thigh bone is broken!" I shouted as I pulled a large splint out of the Unit 1 and taped it tightly around the thigh. Then I pulled a bottle of Ringer's and started an IV on him. It blew my mind how these kids could ignore pain. The only way he would have recognized the problem would have been when the thing fell off. Had he walked any longer on that fracture, it would have ripped his femoral artery and he would have bled out on me in minutes. I was mad at the kid for not caring enough about his own body to let me take care of him satisfactorily.

"Don't you move that leg one inch! You can bleed out in minutes if that broken bone cuts your big artery down there. Don't you move, no matter what happens. I'll take care of everything."

"Yes sir." That was it. I lost my cool. I shouted loud enough so all the conscious men in the chopper belly could hear, "Goddamn it, let's get this straight. I'm a doctor, not an officer. I'm your doctor, not your commander. Don't call me 'sir.'"

"Yes sir, I mean yes, doctor."

"And furthermore, you are not a Marine now. You're a sick patient. Now stop being such a goddamn macho he-man and start worrying about yourself. Start worrying about your own body. Pay attention to pain. If you don't, you're gonna kill yourself."

"Yes, doctor." He burst into tears, shaking his head. I felt like shit. This was no time to give sermons. Some beliefs should be kept silent.

I returned to the men on the litters. The guy with the flank wound was turning ashen, his pulse was weak and thready, his respiration shallow. I checked the IV – open and running at full speed. I checked the ABD pad: dry. I felt the belly – soft. He was losing blood pressure. His pulse became weaker, his breathing shallower. He was losing blood volume. I had to do something. There was no more Ringer's Lactate, so I ripped a bottle of albumin off the strap of the Unit 1 bag, jabbed the needles in the bottle and then jabbed the needle into a large vein on his other arm.

Thank God I got to him before his circulation collapsed!

I set the flow to maximum. Shortly after the flow of albumin started, the pulse became stronger for a minute or two, then became weak and thready again, and within five minutes it stopped.

The crew chief and I began to perform cardiopulmonary resuscitation.

When the chopper landed at Charlie Med, a fresh group of corpsmen jumped in to spare us, but it was futile. Even one of the doctors from Charlie Med boarded the chopper to see if he could do anything. He saw the situation was hopeless and quietly sat down on the sling seat, shaking his head in frustration. I sat down next to him.

"I'm Al Levin. I just started here as new flight surgeon at Dong Ha."

"I'm Dan O'Brien. I've been here at Charlie Med for six months. I've seen too much of this carnage."

"I'm fresh to the job and it's too much for me."

"FNG? You poor sucker! This place will drive you nuts."

There they were. The same words Dan was using, Art had too. Was I to be driven crazy by my experiences here? Nobody seemed to question it. It was just a matter of fact… and of time.

Did I Screw Up?

"Hey Dan," I asked, turning my head from the carnage in front of us, "I had Ringer's Lactate running at full bore on him and his blood pressure still dropped out on me. I got a little spurt with the albumin, but it seemed to be too late. What do you think happened?"

"Al, these wounds are nothing like you'll ever see in civilian life. It's bizarre. I did my orthopedic surgery residency at NYU and rotated through Bellevue's emergency room for years. I never saw wounds like these. These are healthy, athletic kids who are quite strong. In combat their adrenals have been pumping at maximum capacity for days at a time. They ignore pain. These kids keep humping until they blow out.

Managing bleeding in a shock trauma victim in the civilized world compared to here is like a car tire with a slow leak and one that blows out at ninety miles an hour. Back home, Ringer's and saline are perfectly good plasma expanders. Even here at Charlie Med, where we can surgically go in after bleeders and give Decadron and Mannitol IV and they're all right. But in the field, albumin is better. We seem to have much better luck keeping the blood pressure up. It keeps the fluids in the veins better."

"Luck!" I cried, "Do you think we could have saved that guy if I'd first used albumin?"

"I don't know. We don't know why he dropped his pressure. We'll never know. If this were the States, we could do an autopsy and find out. Not in this hell hole," he pronounced as he stood up to leave.

"Did I screw up?"

Dan stopped and turned back to me. "Al, you're going to lose a lot of guys out here. Some of these guys are not salvageable. This place is insane – absolutely mindless chaos and butchery. Don't blame yourself. What we are doing is all new. Never before have we been able to get to wounded soldiers so soon after they've been wounded. In other wars, most of these guys would have died before the doctors got to them. We're just learning how to deal with these problems. If you blame yourself for making mistakes, you'll be ineffectual and of no help to anyone. These guys will die, and sometimes there will be nothing you can do about it. Remember that. I've got to go now. Good luck."

Sitting on my seat, flying back to Dong Ha, I still questioned my-self.

Could I have saved that man with albumin?

Did we lose him because I used Ringer's Lactate first?

That was an eighteen-year-old kid!

Somebody's son?

Brother?

High school sweetheart?

Did we lose him because I screwed up?

No Action Last Night

One morning, I awoke in a daze. Did I sleep all night? No mortar attacks? I asked myself hopefully –

Maybe things are slowing down?

Finally rested and undistracted, I noticed just how slimy my rat-infested bunker was and how filthy I was. As usual, I'd slept in my flak jacket, underwear, and combat boots. I had weeks of stubble on my face and an itchy rash from body lice. My crotch was raw and the skin burned from dried sweat, piss, and fecal matter. My feet were blistered with a chronic fungal infection.

How was I still even walking?

With the lull, I figured it was safe enough to clean myself up. I had to be very careful removing my boots and socks. Any further damage to my skin could make the infection worse. I could wind up in the hospital for IV antibiotics and systemic fungal medications.

Hold on just a second.

A couple of weeks laying up in bed? Three squares a day? No bullets zipping by?

Out of this shitstorm?

It was sure tempting, but I never was much of a malingerer. After removing my socks, I poured a canteen of fresh water over my feet and dried them.

Clean enough, I guess.

Donning my grimy flight suit, I picked up my flak jacket, helmet, Unit 1, rifle, .38, and cartridge belt, having decided to walk over to the operations bunker complex. Major Schneider was there with several of the pilots.

"What's happening?" I asked.

"It's active in western I Corps. Hard getting in. Lots of rain forest with heavy jungle canopy. No LZs. No clear roads. We're having to air drop supplies to the troops, and any Medevacs will have to be hoisted into the chopper," he explained.

Hate Those Hoists

"Sounds like fun," I replied. "I'll get my corpsman to set up the stretchers."

For a moment, my thoughts drifted off to Pensacola and a warm sparkling afternoon training session on helicopter hoists. The stretchers were wire frame litters. The wounded were strapped in and lifted up to the chopper. This wasn't too bad in the UH-34s because they had a wide door to bring the litter aboard. The tricky hoist was into the CH-46s, as I had remembered from training. You had to tilt the stretcher a little from the horizontal in order to get it through the chopper's belly hatch.

When I walked into the Medevac hootch, I interrupted Frank playing acey ducey with one of the chopper crew chiefs. "Hey Frank," I called, "did you hear that we're going to have to do some stretcher hoists?"

"Really, Doc? I hate those fuckin' hoists. There you are with your ass hangin' in the breeze, just waitin' for the gooks to take a pot shot at you." All of a sudden, I realized this wasn't going to be like in training. Now they'd be shooting at us!

Frank and I walked over to the airstrip where we stored the stretchers. We pulled out two in order to check their straps and fasteners. Frank began grumbling, "I'd sure feel like shit if I strapped a grunt into one of these things and he got shot or fell out on the way up to the chopper."

"Has that ever happened?"

"I don't know, don't remember hearing about that around here," he replied, "but I don't think we've really done that many."

"Let's triple check everything and practice," I suggested.

We checked. They were sound, so we grabbed one of them and

loaded it into the UH-34D designated as the Medevac bird for our flight. We placed the other stretcher behind the operations bunker, just in case we needed it.

That morning remained peaceful. Frank took the single priority Medevac which was a soldier with high fever and severe diarrhea who needed to be moved to Charlie Med where he could be treated with antibiotics and IV fluids. Frank didn't need the stretcher we'd gotten out.

But, it wasn't quiet for long.

WHOP-WHOP-WHOP

Then the call… *Emergency Medevac!*

From the operations bunker, Larry Hurley, the radio operator yelled, "Two grunts tripped a bouncing betty and survived. It's not hot right now. But they're down in a canyon under thick canopy. Here's your hoist."

At least there were no reports of combat activity in the area, but that could easily change.

"You can never tell," Schneider warned. "The gooks can set up an ambush in the hills. Since they know the chopper will have to dip into the canyon for a hoist, they can take the high ground on either side of the canyon and have an ideal firing position at the chopper."

"I got it, Doc," Frank hollered as he ran to the chopper. No need for me to go.

"Good luck, man. Sounds like a tough one." I replied, trying to empathize with him. I watched as the Medevac flight took off for the hills, then went into the operations bunker to monitor the radio calls. Things remained quiet for the first few minutes, then we heard Barney Whalen shouting over the radio, "We're takin' rounds from the north. Come in to cover us."

"We got 'em," replied a Huey pilot.

"We're out of control! We've got to cut!" came Barney's frantic voice. Then silence. My gut wrenched and I got the dry heaves. Ten minutes later, we are relieved by the welcome sound of the chopper's radio and their approach. Gazing into the sky, I expected to see three birds, but counted all four aircraft from that mission, which was un-usual because one should have split off to take the wounded man to the hospital.

Something was terribly wrong. I ran to the chopper and looked into the belly. Frank, the gunner and the crew chief sat there stunned.

"What happened?" I hollered.

"We lowered the stretcher into the jungle," shouted Frank. "The corpsmen below strapped the grunt in and signaled for us to hoist him up. Just as we were straining to pull the stretcher through the trees, we started taking rounds. One hit the windscreen, and I guess the pilot jerked around to avoid more hits. That started the stretcher in a wild rotation and before we knew it, the thing was swinging out below, pulling us out of the sky. We had to cut it loose. The guy must have flown a quarter of a mile before he crashed into the hillside. What a goddamn mess!"

"Holy shit!" I replied. "We've got to come up with something better."

Crafting a Safer Stretcher

With the choppers refueled and shut down, Frank, Barney, and I went to the operations bunker to discuss the horrible mishap. "How come that doesn't happen when we're using the horse collar for lifting?" I asked.

'That's because you're lifting in the vertical position," answered Schneider. "These litters are horizontal. They set up a sympathetic rotation in the opposite direction from the rotor blades."

"What about those canvas litters they use aboard ship to haul guys vertically through hatches?" I asked. "Why don't we use those?"

"They're not strong enough for airborne, long-distance hoists," Schneider glumly explained.

"What if we make them stronger?" I asked. "Can we get one?"

"They've got to have some on the *Repose*," Barney volunteered, referring to the USS Repose hospital ship. "I'll have one brought in when they Medevac someone out there, no later than tomorrow morning."

Sure enough that next morning, in the operations bunker, I found a new rescue stretcher, originally designed in the early 1900s, and modified over time. It was made of heavy canvas, shaped like the contour of the body with two flaps and straps that covered the chest and two that covered the lower trunk and legs.

The boys were right. This stretcher which had Velcro fasteners was not strong enough to safely use in a combat flight operation. I knew that with the severe vibrations and significant swaying of a chopper, the fasteners wouldn't safely hold the weight of a human body.

Easy enough, I thought. *Strengthen the straps.*

On the stretcher, I fashioned a series of heavy-duty four-inch-wide canvas cargo straps fastened with steel snaps, which I placed in strategic areas perpendicular to the longitudinal axis of the stretcher – two crossed the chest, one went around the waist, one across the thighs, one over the knees, and one across the ankles. For over the forehead, I fashioned a broad canvas sheet that would restrain the head of an unconscious man during the hoist. Having all of the straps in place, I kept them in place temporarily with adhesive tape. The next step was to firmly stitch the straps to the canvas litter. That meant shipping everything off to the parachute shop at the Danang Air Base, with specific instructions as to what I wanted. So, I rolled up the stretcher and straps, placed them aboard a resupply chopper returning to Marble Mountain and radioed the parachute fitter. Four hours later, I got it

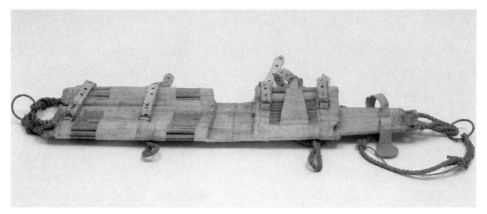

Image of stretcher used in rescue hoists of the wounded, modified by Lt. Levin and adopted for widespread use by the U.S. Marines (Source: U.S. Navy)

back, all stitched and ready for testing. I grabbed it and ran to the operations bunker.

"Frank," I shouted excitedly, "I think we've got the problem licked."

"Yeah, Doc," he chortled. "You're gonna make 'em flyin' mummies."

"Just about, man, just about. Come here and look at this. What do you think?"

Frank examined the contraption. "Will it hold a fat guy like me?"

"Let's try!" I opened it up and readied it for him.

All that evening and into the night, Frank and I worked on the stretcher – trying to rip it apart, hoisting it repeatedly on a parked chopper. That next day, we took our testing up a notch. With the chopper flying in a low hover, I had Frank strap me in the stretcher as we performed a hoist. It all checked out. We were ready.

That's good because later that morning, we got the chance to try the new modifications in action.

Field Testing Our Newly Modified Hoist

"Medevac! Medevac!"

"We have a grunt with a bad gut wound," hollered the radio operator. "They think they got all the gooks, so the area should be quiet".

"Let me take this one. I want to test the stretcher," I said.

"Damn it, Doc! Quit grandstandin'," Frank hollered. "You don't know this will be quiet. Why don't we wait for an easier run?"

"I appreciate the concern, Frank, but I'll be okay."

"You just watch your butt, Doc. I can be replaced real easy. You can't."

"Frank, almost nothing I've done in this shitty war has required a medical degree. At this rate I could be replaced by an orangutan," I retorted as I gathered all of my gear and ran off toward the waiting chopper.

As we lifted off, I hollered to the crew chief, "We're testing out a new stretcher for hoisting. I'll carry it down to the zone in the horse collar and strap the grunt in, then you hoist the litter up and in and lower the line for me. Tell the pilots what we're doing." He gave me the thumbs up signal and began talking over the intercom. At one point he shrugged his shoulders and shook his head. Then he nodded. "What did they say?" I shouted.

"They said the Doc must be out of his fuckin' gourd," he answered with a smile.

"So what else is new?" I replied.

We reached the drop zone in less than fifteen minutes and established a hover. Among the trees we could make out the wounded man on a bright orange tarpaulin surrounded by a number of grunts, two of whom stood by him to assist in the hoist operation. I donned the horse collar, grabbed the stretcher, locked and loaded my M-14 and gave the crew chief the thumbs up.

Slowly, they lowered me through the belly hatch and down under the chopper. I noticed a very slow spin, but since the 46 had tandem counter rotating blades, there was no marked sympathetic rotation. The spin allowed me to get a good view of the surrounding terrain. With the stretcher in my left arm and the rifle in my right, I hung from the horse collar like a paratrooper in harness.

On the ground I quickly detached the horse collar from the drop line and attached the litter, then had the two grunts attending the wounded man lift him onto it. After being sure the ABD pad on his belly was secure, I strapped him tightly in, gave the thumbs up signal to the crew chief and watched as the litter slowly rose towards the chopper.

The crew chief easily recovered the stretcher and within moments I saw the line coming back down. To give it weight, it had an ammo box attached. When I got a hold of it, I detached the ammo box, hooked up my horse collar, waved goodbye to the grunts, gave the crew chief the signal, and up I went, too elated to think of the danger of being shot while dangling from the line.

When I boarded the chopper without difficulty, everyone let out a cheer, and even the wounded grunt had a big smile on his face. I got the stretcher unfastened and an IV of albumin going within minutes. We dropped the grunt off at Charlie Med with no problems.

The truth is, we were ecstatic.

From then on, we used the new stretcher for all our litter hoists. My commanding officer submitted the design to the U.S. Marine high command and it became standard equipment.

I quietly bragged on myself –

Leave it to a Jewish boy with our learned propensity to earnestly question, even rebel, seeking better alternatives.

By God, we're creative innovators!

Doctors of Battlefield Medicine

Innovating on the fly was certainly required on this typical hot and muggy day, where the humid air wrapped around you like cellophane and was full of hungry mosquitoes. Distracting us from our physical misery, came the familiar roar of *WHOP-WHOP-WHOP*, faint at first and slowly amplifying. Then, the strident call, "Medevac! Medevac!"

I knew they'd need me.

My body automatically set out at a dead run. My conscious mind followed. Boarding the chopper, I was toting my typical gear – cement shirt, flak jacket, helmet, M-14, .38, survival knife, ass insurance and my Unit 1 with five bottles of albumin taped to the strap and plastic fuel pipe that I carried to use for either a tracheostomy or chest tube as needed.

I can barely breathe.

I'm so goddamn tired.

How the hell can I just keep going?

As I hurled myself aboard the chopper, we began our take-off run. With his communications line to the pilot, the crew chief was advised as to the nature of the Medevac and leaned over to shout at me, "This one's an emergency, Doc. We've got a grunt that caught one in the face."

Now, a face wound could mean any one of a number of things, as this information had come to us second-hand through a grunt medic to a radioman, or possibly even from one of the combat infantrymen.

Therefore, my two major considerations involved reducing bleeding and maintaining an airway.

If I needed to do a tracheostomy, I would fashion a makeshift tube out of six inches of the plastic fuel pipe I always brought along. I never bothered to carry the ordinary tracheostomy tubes because, if the wound was bad enough to require tracheostomy, the fuel pipe would be more than adequate and I wouldn't have to worry about sizes, shapes and maintaining sterility. Besides, the fuel pipe could easily double for a chest tube and in a pinch could even be used as a tourniquet.

With limitations on the amount of material I could physically carry, the fuel pipe afforded far more adaptability and flexibility than specialized pieces of equipment for each separate procedure. Crude but effective in that I only had to maintain the airway for ten to fifteen minutes until the wounded man got to a rear facility where a real tracheostomy could be performed.

Then I broke out a bottle of albumin and hung it on a rack inside the belly of the chopper, attached the plastic tubing, and readied the needle for insertion into a vein. After my first episode with the grunt bleeding out on me, I never bothered to assess the cardiovascular situation of my wounded charge. I always started intravenous albumin. If I did it unnecessarily, it wouldn't hurt, and it could make the difference between life and death.

The chopper began to lurch and shift power in a manner that made me aware we were coming down into heavy combat. Our bird rattled and shuddered and filled with the din of its engines roaring at their highest speed. In an approach that rattled my teeth and shook my innards, we landed hard. In only a few seconds, two Marines brought the wounded man in a modified fireman's carry and just heaved him aboard the chopper, ass-end first.

The poor bastard just skidded in towards us and became my total responsibility since the crew chief and gunner were attentively scanning their areas with their M-60 machine guns. No sooner had they tossed the guy on board than the chopper blades surged, taking sweeping bites of air in order to hurl us out of that hot zone. As we lifted off, we made wild S-turn maneuvers and low-level wing-overs to avoid ground fire. The crew chief and gunner both opened up with their M-60s, showering me with empties.

I focused my attention on the horrible wound before me. The grunt's face was smashed. The entire left side of his jaw was shattered with pieces of his left mandible embedded in the right maxilla behind his teeth. Fortunately, his tongue, though ripped in pieces, only oozed blood. I could see no active bleeders. Because it was dusk and difficult to see, I couldn't ascertain the color of his face. Because of his heaving chest, though, I could tell that he was having difficulty bringing in air. I reached for an airway and tried to jam it around his tongue as he lay there only semi-conscious and thrashing around, but I couldn't get it through. I was just jamming part of his tongue back into his trachea, making matters worse. I had to do something, so I reached my hand into the soggy mess that was all that remained of his mouth, feeling for an opening, but all that did was only push tissue back into his trachea.

Emergency Tracheostomy: Survival Knife and Fuel Pipe

I had only one option – tracheostomy. That was his only chance. I'd practiced for this for months, but I'd never thought I'd have to do it under these horrid conditions. It was too damn dark to reach into my Unit 1 for my scalpel. Besides, I had my survival knife and that was good enough. I always carried my large hemostats attached to the outside of my bag so that if I needed them to stop bleeding, I'd have them immediately.

I straddled the thrashing, wounded Marine, using my knees to pin his elbows. He was fighting me and his chest was heaving, so I knew I only had a few more minutes. With my knife in one hand I felt for his trachea with my other, almost completely in the dark. The chopper heaved and swayed with evasive maneuvers that kept throwing me off balance. Finally identifying his trachea with my left index finger, I carefully slashed at it with my knife. Almost immediately, I could feel the rush of air entering the hole my incision had created. I quickly inserted my hemostat to maintain patency of the hole. Then the Marine relaxed. His breathing became regular.

Thank God! I've gotten that airway open!

Next, I inserted the piece of plastic fuel pipe into the trachea in order to maintain the hole. That proved surprisingly easy. In order to be sure it didn't get sucked into the trachea, I kept my hand over the open end of the plastic pipe. I also wanted to make sure it didn't kink and block his airway. Then I carefully taped the protruding end of the fuel pipe to his neck to keep the passage open until we could get to the hospital.

Once the Marine relaxed and I had an airway again, I could think about his cardiovascular system. Fortunately, he was a muscular guy, and I could feel his large veins, so I immediately started an IV of albumin and gave it to him as fast as I could, then checked his pulse, which was strong enough. I felt that was all I could do for him, periodically checking the end of the fuel pipe to feel the air from his exhaling and inhaling. It was a drastic measure, fraught with all kinds of potential complications, but I knew he would have died without it.

I felt like I'd finally been able to use my medical skills successfully. *You did it, Doc, in the dark, with a knife and fuel hose.*

Letter of Appreciation from the Big Honcho

In April of 1967, I'd been in-country for just a couple of months. A letter of appreciation had arrived for me from Major General L.B. Robertshaw, our Commanding General in the Pacific. Major General L.B. Robertshaw had written to me, a lowly Lieutenant – a reservist and draftee. In the subject was typed: "Letter of Appreciation." It goes

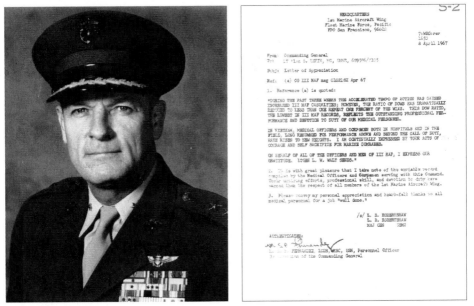

Major Gen. Louis Robershaw USMC Commanding General of the Pacific (Credit: USMC)

on to state:

"During the past three weeks, the accelerated tempo of action has caused increased III MAF casualties. However, the ratio of DOWS (% of deaths following admission to a medical facility) has dramatically reduced to less than 1%. Repeat 1% of the WIAS (wounded in action). This DOW ratio, the lowest in III MAF records, reflects the outstanding professional performance and devotion to duty of our medical personnel. I am continually impressed by your acts of courage and self-sacrifice for Marine comrades."

Sounds really impressive, doesn't it? With me being just a draftee and troublemaker.

Our big honcho was thanking me personally and, of course, my fellow combat medical personnel for saving lives, in performing our duties at the highest performance levels ever achieved. Because of our bravery in the line of fire, more of our Marines would be returning home.

I didn't even read the letter.

Whatever it said, I knew, would only remind me not of the lives we were saving but the senseless loss of the many we could not.

That made me angry.

Chapter Six
Home Unsafe Home

Darkness comes and the clouds turn black with threatening rain.
An eerie feeling creeps into your whole being as the beautiful trees of daytime
turn into laughing demons from the cold night wind.
Sgt. Bruce F. Anello
A Pawn in the Game: A Vietnam Diary
Killed in Action on May 31, 1968

Typically, they'd storm us at night. We called them sappers. These are North Vietnamese army commandos. Many of them are just teenagers, some even in their early teens. They swarm us like ants on a suicide mission to infiltrate our bases, to kill troops and lay charges to blow up aircraft, ammunition dumps, and any other targets of opportunity. If even only some of them are successful, obviously, they wreak havoc. We're attacked and killed right in our own hootches. Sure, we had perimeter defenses, but still rest was fitful, at best. To wear us down, NVA commanders were more than willing to sacrifice however many kamikaze-style fighters necessary to inflict physical and psychological damage on us.

In combat, troops grab sleep wherever and whenever possible. Hopefully, you're successful here and there at catching a few precious hours of genuine slumber. Even a few minutes, though, is welcome, throwing a partial charge on your battery. That's one of the basic axioms on the battlefield – any chance you get to stop moving, then sleep. You have no idea how many hours you'll have to be wide awake defending your position. And when your life depends on it, your fear keeps you alert and even profound exhaustion at bay.

We were always afraid that sappers would infiltrate our area but felt relatively safe because our hootches stood well within the perimeter. Any invading enemy soldiers would have to get past the boundary guards, then cross the airfield and penetrate the operations area before they got to us. Because the entire area had been sprayed with a defoliant that we were told was harmless, we had wide open views of the areas that surrounded us.

No gook will risk being out in the open with our sights on him.

That's what we thought.

We were wrong.

Since a helicopter squadron is limited in its night operations, we usually bedded down shortly after sundown. On this particular night, it was no different from any other. As a matter of fact, the sky was relatively clear, permeated by brilliant moonlight, which would in most circumstances indicate that the enemy would stay away. It would be fairly easy to sight them and mount a significant counter-offensive if they attempted to break through our defenses.

I went to sleep on my cot. The sides of our tent were rolled up with our bunkers just a quick roll away. All of our gear was within reach to grab if we had to take cover – flak jacket, helmet and weapons. It wasn't unusual to wake up in your bunker wearing your gear and holding your rifle. You'd gain full consciousness to the crackle of small arms fire or mortar shell explosions shaking the ground around you.

Anyone in combat learns to sleep with their ears tuned – for the unmistakable sign of the mortar shell falling down its tube and striking the firing pin, or the sound of incoming artillery shells before their impact with the ground. In such dire circumstances, the unconscious mind very often drives the body to take remedial actions like donning protective gear and hitting the ground before the conscious mind becomes aware of any of those actions.

Wait, My Hand's Warm

This particular night I will never forget. It still haunts me. I woke up in my bunker, except it wasn't from gunfire and explosions. I was confused. I had my flak jacket and helmet on. I wasn't on my belly but crouching on my knees. Then I realized I was jammed up against something – something over my head – that was pressing down on me. I realized I was pushing it with my arm. My hand was grasping something, something steel, covered with a leather handle. It was my survival knife. It felt good to have that in my hand. It offered protection. However, it was warm.

Wait!

Warm steel?

What's going on?

My hand's warm... and wet.

Warm, wet... and sticky.

Suddenly, I snapped into full consciousness. I felt the handle of my knife throbbing in my hand, ka-lump, ka-lump, ka-lump. And I heard the agonized groan of a small man. I'd stabbed him.

Feeling His Dying Fibrillation

Only then did I grasp that I had surprised a gook climbing into my hole and I had hit him right in the gut with my knife. I'd thrust it into his solar plexus, upward through his diaphragm and into his left ventricle. It had been his heartbeat, and then his dying fibrillation that I'd felt, while blood poured out of his chest over my knife, over my hand, my arm and my entire right shoulder, as his limp body slid down over my back like a sack of potatoes.

Then and only then, I realized the stark terror of hand-to-hand combat. I awoke fully to the utter chaos when enemy soldiers successfully invade your base and home.

I could hear my buddies shouting to one another, "They're overrunning us! They're overrunning us!" I bolted up out of my hole and started running at top speed towards the Marine infantry division camped about a quarter mile behind us because I knew I'd have much more protection with combat soldiers around. As I ran I knew that I would be an easy target, so I began weaving around so that if anybody tried to get the bead on me, at least he'd have a hard time hitting me.

I didn't have very far to run, a hundred yards or so, when I saw the guys had already assembled and formed a potent defensive boundary, all lined up with their automatic weapons, their M-60 machine guns, and the tanks which had begun to roll in our direction.

"Come over here, Doc!" One of the grunts called out. I ran in his direction and leapt over the sandbag wall head-first into his hole, did a somersault and ended sitting up, half dazed and utterly terrified. I still had my bloody knife in my hand. I was sweaty, sticky and stinking.

The grunt asked, "You okay, Doc?"

"I don't know. I think so."

"What happened?"

"I guess I got some young gook when he was trying to crawl into my hole. All I know is that I was asleep and then I was awake with my knife in his guts. Bastard bled all over me. Hope he doesn't have hepatitis or syphilis."

"Jesus, Doc. Can't you ever forget medicine?"

"Yeah... Forget medicine... That's what I should do."

After things finally had quieted down, we went back to my tent to see whether the guy was still there. We found no body. Typical of sappers, they had dragged off their fatalities, just as we try not to leave any of ours behind. There was no question the little sapper, just a teenager, was dead, though. I had at least half his blood volume all over me.

Our Killer Quack

From then on, throughout the entire squadron, I gained a new nickname –

"Killer Quack"

With comedic glee, my buddies presented me a special coffee mug they'd sent off for, with that title emblazoned on its side.

One hell of a moniker!

I wondered what Hippocrates would have said about this distinction. After some days of uncomfortable amusement, I asked the guys whether they could find it in their hearts to provide me with a less lethal-sounding tribute. They sent away again to their mail order source and presented me with a replacement mug that to this day sits on the shelf above my desk. In its gold filigree it proclaims, much more innocuously, "Flight Quack."

That, I liked.

Hell Raining Down

Besides the invasions and waking up having to fight hand to hand to the death, we lived with the constant fear of being blown up during one of the ongoing bombardments. Day and night, our bases along the DMZ got hammered with rocket, artillery and mortar barrages.

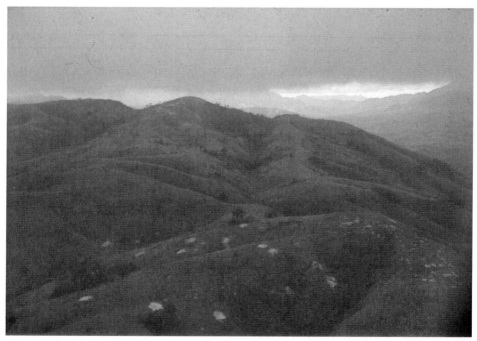

Aerial view of light-colored impact craters left by exploding ordinance (Credit: Dave Petteys)

Flying into Dong Ha or other U.S. bases, you notice the landscape is littered with distinct white patches. Those are craters left by exploding ordinance, fired from enemy positions, trying to weaken our capability to support military operations along the DMZ. This was especially true in the Khe Sanh area, where a big battle was being anticipated.

Once, I spent 10 hours straight in my bunker as hell rained down, the explosions – direct hits and misses – the sheer terror of not knowing if you were going to be blasted to pieces. It was like being trapped in a treacherous thunderstorm, with lightning strikes occurring around you.

Am I next?

In his book, *Marine Helo*, Petteys describes a rocket and mortar attack on Dong Ha, as the First Battle for Khe Sanh had gotten underway: "April 28, 1967: At 2:50 A.M., we were awoken by a series of violent explosions. Shrapnel was raining down on the roof. Naked and barefoot, I leaped into my sandbag bunker. I felt helpless. What if we took a direct hit? How long will it last? I am shaking like a leaf and

I feel sick. When it was over, we suffered some 20 casualties and 50 wounded. One poor devil was killed in bed. Then, his hooch burned. What a sight!"

Such attacks are like a ticket to a live horror movie. However, this action thriller was for keeps.

When the artillery attacks started, we'd hear a series of sharp popping sounds that reached us from what seemed to be far away. Suddenly, we get rocked with what sounded like freight trains overhead.

KABOOM!

Everything slows down.

There is almost no noise, just a faint, powerful whooshing sound. I felt like I was being tightly squeezed. All of the screens on the hootch blew in, and a fine cloud of dust rose in the air. Everyone seemed to stand still, frozen in place. I could see my buddies' clothes compress against their skin as if they were submerged under water.

Then, everything snapped back to normal speed, and I heard "Incoming! Incoming artillery!" And the sirens began to blare as the air filled with the sound of explosions and concussions. The closer the shells hit, the greater the strength of the blast shockwave.

KABOOM!

KABOOM!

"All planes airborne! Scramble! Scramble!" Schneider shouted. "All ground personnel in the bunkers on the double!"

The pilots and flight crews rushed to the aircraft and got off the ground in minutes. I ran for the nearest bunker about fifty feet down from the ready room hootch, dived in headfirst, curled into the far corner with my back to the wall, and covered my head with my arms. The explosions continued, with the concussions not so intense now that I was below ground level. The shells continued to pour into the compound, with each explosion preceded by a popping sound followed by the roar of an airborne freight train.

"Loosen up, Doc. It'll be over in a few minutes," came a comforting voice from the other side of the bunker, where Gunnery Sergeant Wallace hunkered down. Gunny Wallace was an old salt. He'd fought in Korea and had spent his first tour in Vietnam with an infantry battalion. He didn't seem overly rattled.

"You're safe here from everything but a direct hit, and there ain't

116

no position you can take to protect yourself from that." I felt a bit more confident.

"Besides," he continued, "you ought to be looking at the entrance with your rifle ready for any gooks who may try to lob a grenade in here. Sometimes they hit one side of a camp with arty or mortars and try an overrun on the other."

"Jesus, do you ever get used to this stuff?"

"No," he chuckled. "You never do. You can't take nothin' for granted in combat. Soon's you do, you're dead."

"How did you get to know all of this?"

"You'll get to know these things, too. It all comes natural. You get to know the difference between the muzzle report of the 15 and the mortar tubes blown'. You'll know the difference in your sleep. It'll come to you naturally. You'll be in a hole before the first shell hits the ground. It'll be part of your life, or you won't make it. You won't forget it, either." He concluded with wry smile.

"I remember way back to Korea. It don't change. It's all the same. My gunny in Korea went through the South Pacific in World War Two. He said it was the same. War don't change. The only way you can help yourself in this bunker is to keep your rifle on the entrance."

I did just that.

Feeling the cold metal barrel of my M-14, I checked to be sure the clip was full, locked it in, loaded the chamber, and sat with the muzzle pointed at the entrance. That made me feel better. Even though it was obvious that the rifle shell was no match for the artillery, I felt protected and invulnerable. After seemingly endless minutes of the enemy's intense bombardment, the frequency of the popping sounds from launching cannons diminished and the airborne freight trains of incoming shells became less frequent. Yet I was confused. There continued to be as many, if not more, huge explosions occurring on our base, but concentrated.

"What's going on?" I asked the gunny, feeling really uneasy.

"I don't know yet," he replied. Now, looking worried.

Our Ammo Dump Just Blew

On September 3, 1967, we'd gotten hit really hard.

"They got the ammo dump!" a voice from outside shouted. "Stay in the bunkers!"

"Do you think any of our guys are caught above ground and wounded?" I called out.

"Doc, don't worry about it. Besides, no way you can get to them now. Just relax. There'll be plenty to do when this quiets down," whoever it was reassured me.

Despite his attempt to sound calm and comforting, I detected a note of agitation. I knew, deep down, he was as terrified as I was. Interspersed with the explosions of the larger shells, we could hear rounds of small arms firing off.

"The small arms ammo and the rockets are cookin' now!" the gunny exclaimed. "If the fire gets to the central bunker, we'll hear the 155s go off."

"Wonder what's going to be left of Dong Ha when this is over?"

"Yeah, me too." The gunny's tone betrayed anger. "I just got me a new stereo outfit on R&R. Goddamn gooks probably destroyed it by now."

As the base exploded and burned, we sat in the damp, cool bunker trying to make ourselves as comfortable as possible. An acrid smoke cloud smelling of burned wood, fuel oil, and gunpowder settled over us. I tried to relax, but my flight suit was soaked and my body as stiff as a two by four.

"Hey, Gunny," I asked, trying to make small talk, "how come the gooks have 15s and we have 155s for artillery shells?"

"We got NATO standardized ammo. That means all NATO countries can use the same ammo – 7 mm rifle shells, 155 mm artillery shells. The gooks have the commie crap – they call it Warsaw Pact. That's 7.25 mm rifle shells and 151 arty. I guess that's so if one guy overruns the other, he can't use his ammo."

Clever, I mused. Both sides have been preparing for this thing for years. Wonder why nobody clued me in on it so I could have figured out some way to avoid this hellhole? Hours passed as the explosions and fire continued.

"I'm gonna look out and see if I can see anything," the sergeant told me as he peeked through the bunker's door.

"Careful, man! There's still a lot of shit going on out there," I hollered to him.

Everything's On Fire

"Man!" he exclaimed, ducking back into the bunker. "The whole base is burnin'! Everything's on fire! What a fuckin' mess!"

The sergeant sat down again, fidgeting. He looked at me with soulful eyes, face filled with guilt. "Doc, I got to piss. I've been holdin' it for hours, but I can't no longer."

"Go ahead, man. It can't make this bunker any more uncomfortable," I reassured him.

"I'll dig a little hole against this far wall and piss in it so it don't run down on us." He scooped away at the mud, then urinated. The smell of urine mingled with the cloud of gunpowder in the bunker's putrid air.

I tried to remain calm, but the long wait generated more and more panic welling up in my chest. All I wanted to do was get out of that bunker and run. Anywhere. Consciously, I knew that would be silly, even fatal. Unconsciously, I felt like a gutter rat, trapped in a hole with fire all around me. The instinctual, subhuman desire to flee welled up. I successfully suppressed the feeling by grasping and hugging my rifle, even found myself kissing and sucking on its cold metal chamber.

Here I am, a nice Jewish doctor, sucking on a rifle like it was my mother's tit.

And, I was bottle fed!
I don't know what my mother's tit tasted like.
Well, for damn sure it wasn't gun grease.

All Clear, Watch Out for Duds

Looking up from my musings, I saw the gunny sitting across from me with his rifle in his lap and his face pointing towards the entrance. He was snoozing.

If he can do that, maybe we're safe.
For now.

An hour and a half or more passed before the chaos finally died down and everyone at the base began to stir. "All clear! All clear! Watch out for duds," came the call from a nearby bunker. Everyone began to mill around, to assess the damage, which was incredible – everything was collapsed and burned – all of the hootches down in the living area, the metal on the cots' frames was bent, their springs melted, all of the wood and fabric burned. Spent shells lay everywhere. The chow hall, the shitters, the shower hootch – all completely destroyed.

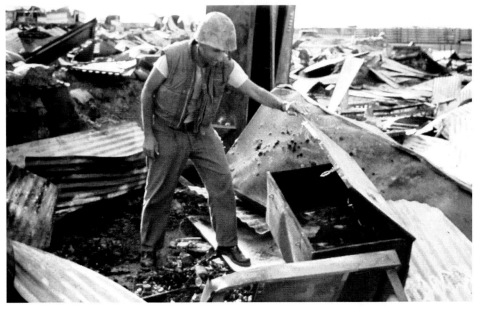

Lt. Al Levin inspecting damage from rocket attack at Dong Ha base, resulting in near total destruction (Credit: Levin Archive)

I ran to Alpha Med, or what was left of it, to handle the casualties. One of the battalion medical officers met me outside of the bunker that served as their medical facility. "How many have we got?" I asked with a sense of foreboding.

"So far, only four dead, all in one hootch. We're seeing a few cuts and bruises and an occasional minor burn, but it looks like we're not going to see anything more serious," he responded.

"You mean to say after all that, we lost only four guys?"

That's incredible! I thought.

"Seems that way, man. Somebody up there likes us," he responded.

"Well, I wouldn't go so far as to say that now," I retorted. "I'm going back to the air wing compound. Send somebody over if you need help later."

As I turned to run back to that part of the compound, I noticed three Marine Corps C-130s landing on the airstrip. Apparently, they had been orbiting over the base until things quieted down. They'd gotten clearance after the runway had been inspected, and in they came.

When I arrived, I stopped Staff Sergeant Gallager and asked: "Did we take any casualties here?"

"No, Doc, not a one, not a one. We only have major damage to one chopper that was stuck on the ground. We were mighty lucky," he said.

"It's great to see those C-130s landing. Amazing they can come in now," I opined.

"Doc, those pilots can land them planes in a cow pasture filled with potholes. You should see them coming into Khe Sanh. Right now for us, they're loaded with C-rations, sleeping bags, and tents so we can begin the cleanup."

Over at the now-leveled communications hootch, the guys were already setting up new radio equipment and maps in the midst of the excavation. A group of infantry officers had come to convene. "The gooks have arty in the DMZ, they have a bead on us, and they'll be lobbing shells in regularly. We're ordering out arc light bombing raids to blow them to kingdom come, but in the meantime we live in bunkers," the captain in the group told everyone.

Over at one of the C-130s, Frank Miller was already unloading medical supplies into a jeep. "Hey Frank, whose wheels?" I hollered.

"I don't know. For now it's ours. I'll put it back when we're through," he snickered.

"Where are we going to set up our operation?" I wondered.

"The guys are digging you a nice bunker, boss. It'll double as our dispensary. We thought you wouldn't mind," he answered.

"No. I always like to live close to my job. I hate commuting to work," commenting as if a little joking might relieve things a bit.

We finished loading the gear and drove to the site of the old dispensary, now blown down and burned out. Just in front of its rubble ten guys were just finishing the new installation – a hole in the ground about four feet deep and ten feet square around the rim of which they'd erected a three-foot-high wall of sandbags stacked so as to create two window spaces on each wall. For front and back entrances, they'd made rampways with steps dug into the dirt and covered by boards. About four feet in front of each entrance stood a double wall of sandbags parallel to the opening that would stop shrapnel from a shell that hit outside the entrance.

"Welcome to your new home, Doc," Frank offered as we drove up.

"Hey Frank, I sure like the skylight!" pointing to the absence of a roof. "But don't you think it'll get a little wet when it rains?"

"Don't worry. These guys know what they're doin'." Just then a six-by truck rolled up, and the guys unloaded twelve-foot long boards, four by eight thick, and a bunch of thick tin panels. Within minutes, they had a solid sandbagged roof on the bunker. They then spread out three or four ponchos on its top and put large rocks on them to keep them down. That was the waterproofing. They had completed the whole structure in a couple of hours.

That what Marines do... for each other.

Oorah!!

Our B-52s Are Coming

Wrapping up our inspection, Charlie Pitman came around. "Looks good, Doc. You'll sleep safe and sound here. By the way, don't worry about the bombing tonight. That's our guys. Our Air Force buddies will operating arc light raids. That outta chase Charlie out of the neighborhood."

"I heard that earlier. What are light raids?" I inquired.

"Carpet bombing missions by B-52's at twenty thousand feet, though it'll sound like they're right overhead. They'll pass just north of the Dong Ha River and lay a carpet of big bombs in a strip half a mile wide and twenty miles long. The ground'll shake, but they'll be far enough away that you can sit on top of the bunker and watch 'em."

Sure enough, that night the rumble of bombers rattled me awake. Pretty soon, just as Charlie had said, the ground began to shake with the fury of the bombardment. Initially, I felt more secure in the bunker, but after realizing that the activity was miles away, I climbed out onto the roof to watch, clad only in my marine green undershorts and combat boots. All of the other guys in the squadron were already on the tops of their bunkers, watching the display and cheering like at a football game.

Horizon on Fire

As each aircraft dropped a line of bombs, the entire horizon would light up brilliantly. First, we'd see bright orange balls erupting sequentially in a forward-moving line. As the explosion matured, the orange would turn to a brilliant white that lit up our camp with what seemed like intense moonlight. Seconds later, we'd hear the intense roar and feel the ground shake from the furious explosions. As those white balls dimmed, another aircraft would drop its load and the light show would start all over again.

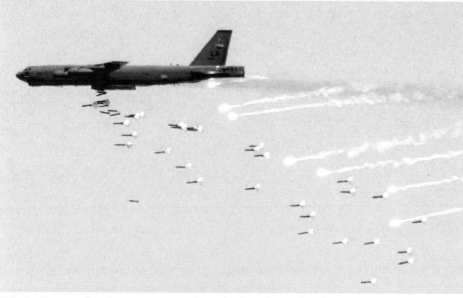

U.S. B-52 carpet bombing mission with its shock and awe (Credit: USAF)

When our brilliant fireworks display seemed to be over, the guys started filtering back down to their bunkers. That's when we heard the now-familiar popping sounds of the 151 muzzle reports followed by the roar of airborne freight trains.

"Incoming! Incoming!" a voice shouted as we all dived into our bunkers.

About a dozen incoming artillery rounds hit in rapid succession about a quarter of a mile to the west of us. Hunched down in my bunker, I listened intently. This time I was prepared. This time I felt protected by the cold steel of the rifle. It wasn't so bad. I could deal with that. The barrage ended in less than five minutes. I waited two or three minutes before I ventured out of my hole, garbed in helmet, flak jacket, rifle, Unit 1, combat boots and green undershorts. "Anybody hurt?" I hollered like a fishmonger in the street.

"None here," came the cry from one area.

"None here," from somewhere else.

"No one here," Miller hollered from his bunker.

"I guess the gooks just want us to know that the B-52s didn't hurt them. They're dug in too well for those bombs to do much damage," said McAllister from the roof of his bunker.

"Shit, Doug," I responded in frustration, "Does that mean we have to live like goddamn moles around here?"

"I guess it does, Doc. I guess it does." His voice trailed off.

Mortared While Intoxicated

On November 10, 1967, celebrating the USMC's 190th birthday, we were in Chu Lai, away from the front, where a group of us were able to finally relax. We were all set up to really indulge ourselves. There hadn't been any activity for three days! It was definitely time to let loose.

It was a beautiful evening. The beer was cold. The char-broiled steaks were scrumptious, char-broiled by the gunny over a make-shift grill, fashioned out of a 55-gallon barrel and metal grate. We kicked back for a few blessedly tranquil hours with Jack, Charley, Ray, and Barry, all plopped down talking about food and women, while a couple of beers had turned me, a recent virtual teetotaler, three sheets to the wind. We drank, ate and laughed, listening to the Mamas and the Papas singing about California dreamin'. It was almost normal.

We were all homesick!

When the party started breaking up, I walked to my hootch and crashed. Finally, a bit of bliss after being in this hellhole for seven goddamn months. I passed out in my bed and having eased off into a comfortable slumberland.

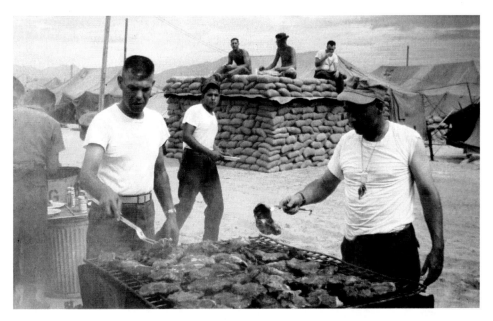
Troops relax with steaks on the 55-gallon drum grill while other grunts are perched on a nearby bunker (Credit: USMC)

Suddenly, I awoke.

What was that?

Where am I?

What's going on?

Again, I had been rattled awake. I was in my foxhole, my helmet on, my flak jacket on, my M-14 at the ready, I heard mortar rounds and felt the concussion of closer impacts as I tasted the sand in my mouth.

BOOM!

BOOM!

BOOM!

Wow. That one was close!

Christ, we're under mortar attack!

They're cross-firing from multiple directions.

Shit!

God, I'm scared.

We were trapped. I was sure stone-cold sober now.

"Doc!"

"Doc!! It's a direct hit! Doc, we need you!"

Shit, they need me.

I don't make house calls!
"Doc! Doc!"
I tried to crawl over to them.
Then, *BOOM!!!*
Shit!
Wow, that was even closer.
What the hell am I doing?

Scurrying across the ground, I came upon three guys. One of them had a stump for a leg, but it wasn't bleeding. A ripped artery can close itself up and the patient may not bleed out. If it were cut, though, it would continue to bleed. Quickly, I applied a tourniquet to the stump. The other guy just had a wound on his arm, which was bleeding pretty badly, but it wasn't going to be much trouble picking out the shrapnel. And he'd go home – probably had some nerve and tendon damage, but as wounds went around there, he wasn't too bad off. The third guy got just a few scratches. I didn't do much with him.

Is it over? I hoped.

Everything grew quiet. I started hollering for help. "Hey, we need some stretcher bearers. We've got to get these guys out of here. Come on. Get your ass up!"

"Keep your head down, Doc. They're going to start up again."

"Come on! Get your fucking stretchers over here."

"Doc, keep your goddamn head down."

Then —

BOOM.

BOOM.

BOOM.

Goddamn it!

Did you have to be right?

I'm trembling.

At least I'm still alive.

BOOM.

BOOM.

Somebody grabbed me. I was led to the side of a badly wounded soldier. His leg was all mangled.

Oh, boy, this kid is really hurting.

Quickly, I administered a dose of morphine, fifteen milligrams, through a curette jabbed directly through his fatigues. As I expected, the kid calmed down. He lessened his grip on my arm and gave me a thankful gaze. I felt relieved. I felt rewarded. At least I could do something to ease his pain and suffering.

These poor kids out here.

Ripped from their parents and girlfriends.

Dumped in foreign land with a rifle and a few weeks of training!

For fucking what?

Once again, the mortars stopped. After ten minutes or so, everybody started scurrying around. Soon, I saw litter bearers coming up with stretchers to start loading the casualties into Jeeps and taking them to Charlie Med. There were a lot of them. It had been a bad attack we hadn't expected.

They going to need me.

I know it.

Another night without sleep.

Hitching a ride to Charlie Med, our oversized bunker dug into the ground, the medical officers there were already working on casualties, with at least five guys needing emergency life-saving procedures. They wouldn't survive a helicopter trip down to the Danang facility. They might not survive anyway.

I was bringing my wounded who needed immediate surgery. I scrubbed in, if that's what you call it, attempting to become as sterile as possible in a putrid cesspool. My eyes burned from the chlorine in the water. Together with the general surgeon and an orthpod, we did what we could.

'Advanced' Medical Care

In the first operation, all three of us needed to work quickly to save this mangled grunt. I started debriding his back, littered with shrapnel wounds that were bleeding. The orthopedic surgeon worked on his mangled hand. The general surgeon on focused on his flank, attempting to pull large pieces of metal shrapnel out of the area of the kidneys and hoping not to sever a renal artery.

We had to be really careful. He'd lost blood. We didn't have enough replacement for him. We just needed to get him stable enough for transport via chopper to the rear naval support hospital. We were hopeful, but always realistically so in the midst of this constant ever-changing turmoil.

And sure enough, just a few minutes into our operation, we began to hear the sound of mortars dropping once again around the compound. Then the alarm siren started.

Holy shit! We were getting mortared again!

Quickly the operating room emptied of everybody but the patient and the surgeons. Terrified, we all stared at one another momentarily and then went back to our tasks at hand – trying to save these guys.

When things quieted, once again everyone else began to filter back into the operating room. Our scrub nurses now had helmets, flak jackets, and sidearms. The circulating nurses had helmets, flak jackets, M-16 rifles, and bandoliers of ammunition. I tried to interject a little humor into the scene.

"Hey, man, can you get me a sterile helmet?"

The orthopod looked up, truly angry. "Shut up, you asshole!"

The operations were certainly tense as mortars continued dropping all over the place. If one made it through the ceiling, we all knew we'd had it. That tin wouldn't stop an 80 mm mortar shell.

As the orthopod worked on the poor grunt's hand, he hollered to the anesthesiologist, "Hey, Joe, pump some more gas. This guy's waking up."

He looked to the orthopod and asked, "What do you mean?"

"Well, I feel him shaking."

He responded, "That ain't him. That's me."

Then a little laughter rippled nervously through the room.

That last of the barrages lasted about five minutes, although it felt like hours. When the final all clear signal sounded, everybody heaved a sigh of relief. We finished up our major cases and shipped them off. We continued on others that night which were mostly minor procedures, like removing shrapnel. These really didn't have to be done by us at Charlie Med but significantly reduced the pressure on the folks down at the Danang facility.

Shell shock? They got that right.

I am numb.

Always on the Run

With the stresses of war, who wouldn't be crapping their pants. We all were.

For sure, being a U.S. Marine in Vietnam meant you suffered from chronic diarrhea. Its cause was obscure but very likely associated with continuous doses of terrifying anxiety, C-rations that were sixty percent fat, foul drinking water that smelled like a sewer but was "sterilized" with enough bromine to burn its drinkers' eyes, or some bacterium or parasite nasty enough to decimate your digestive tract.

Frequent in the trips to my personal four-holer, while performing my daily elimination, I would often have lengthy philosophical discussions with colleagues, like an ancient Roman orator. On occasion, I could be found expounding on medical treatises while sitting on the throne. Not wanting to waste time at a sick call, several of my buddies would come into the shitter to ask me medical questions while we did our daily duty. One day, as I sat on my hole, one of the pilots opened the door of the shitter and asked, "Hey, doc, what do you do for diarrhea?"

After deliberating for a few seconds on the potential etiologic factors involved in this individual's chief complaint, and evaluating the several therapeutic modalities available to an individual with this type of problem, I looked up to him and answered, "Come on in and sit down."

No battle action then. Just a little (or a lot) of bowel action.

Bronze Star with Valor

Like my fellow Marines, I saw my mission as simply doing the best job I could for the guys that were fighting beside me – to do our job and get everyone home – at least, as many as we could. Back home, my family had fought to survive all of my life. I fought growing up in tough times and won. I'd matured into someone who was quite tenacious, even at bit braggadocios at times, excelling at what I did.

Getting to Harvard, I proved to be a top performer – even under extreme stress and in highly demanding conditions. That's how I had advanced into medical research. That's why I thought they wanted me for their astronaut program.

I was wrong. They chose to sacrifice me and others.

These are my comrades in arms who I'd grown to respect and adore – to give them everything I had – even my life.

Looking from the lofty perches of their cozy headquarters, with their underlings buzzing around addressing their every demand, the Marine brass apparently takes the time to recognize bravery among the military's rank and file. They need to maintain high morale, to keep the forces fighting. They pin medals. They'll attend star-spangled ceremonies and notable funerals. And, they hand out U.S. flags to the families of the fallen.

In my case, for my actions in combat operations, I was awarded a Bronze Star with Valor. Quoting Lt. Gen. V.H. Krulak, Commanding General, Fleet Marine Force, Pacific:

"His close personal contact with the men of his unit and constant concern for their welfare materially increased the effectiveness of the squadron in supporting operations. Lieutenant Levin displayed exceptional courage and composure. His prompt and expert care undoubtedly saved the lives of Marines. Striving to improve both the methods and equipment used to hoist medical evacuees to hovering helicopters Lieutenant Levin regularly tested, under combat conditions, a litter he had modified, being lowered to injured men, quickly administered first aid and utilized his improved litter to successfully lift them to the helicopter with a minimum of discomfort. Continually concerned for the welfare of the Vietnamese, Lieutenant Levin participated in a highly successful Medical Civic Action Program at several orphanages in the Marble Mountain area."

Thank you, but I wasn't in it for the glory. I did it for my buddies.

Actually, at the time, I was intensely angry about what was happening to all of us. In fact, I quit the civic action program because the day after we'd left one of the orphanages, the Viet Cong came in and executed the Catholic nuns and the children.

I didn't give a damn anymore.

I ignored all of my combat citations for decades. Now, I feel perhaps a bit differently. It's still quite difficult for me to read them. It triggers horrific memories that make me physically ill, stressed psychologically and emotionally distraught.

Even today, more than a half-century later, reflecting upon them causes me to weep uncontrollably. I do, however, in honor of my fellow comrades.

The ones still living and breathing.

And those not.

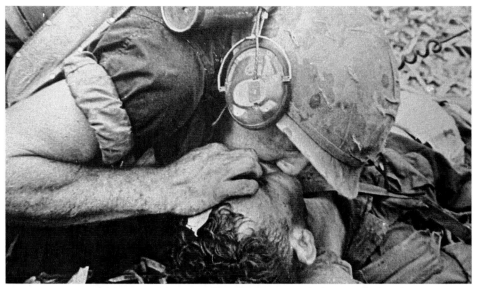

USMC Corpsman delivering life-saving breaths to a wounded comrade (Credit: USMC)

Chapter Seven
Losing Friends and Killing Friendlies

"Hey, Hey LBJ, how many kids did you kill today?"
Protest Chant
1967

Come on wall street don't be slow
Why man this war is a go-go
There's plenty good money to be made by
Supplying the army with the tools of its trade
Let's hope and pray that if they drop the bomb
They drop it on the Viet Cong
And it's one, two, three, what are we fighting for
Don't ask me, I don't give a damn, next stop is Viet Nam
And it's five, six, seven, open up the pearly gates
Ain't no time to wonder why, whoopee we're all gonna die.
County Joe and The Fish
Woodstock Music Festival
1969

One rare lazy afternoon in my hootch, half dozing, I was jolted once again by that noise. That sound. Whop. Whop. Whop. Even today, decades later, it's permanently etched in my mind. I still hear it in my sleep.

Coming into orbit over our airfield were the Hueys from our gunship squadron, accompanied by the familiar cry from the operations officer in the nearby bunker, "Medevac! Medevac!" The raucous commotion drove me out of my sweet state of slumber.

I wasn't thrilled.

I've been asking for a replacement corpsman for days now.
Why can't they send me one?
Damn it!

Our Big Okie

As I leapt into action, I realized something unexpected – a Medevac helicopter was landing at the base. Circling above were their escorts coming back from a mission. Within moments, I was advised that on board was Larry White, one of our corpsmen. He was a big strapping Okie with a shock of dirty blond hair and wide blue eyes, uncomplicated, who never shut up with his incessant fish stories arising out of trips with his father, who was a Marine from World War II. Larry had elected to follow in his footsteps.

Serving as a CH-46A door gunner, Larry's bird was hit with automatic weapons fire from the ground while operating the hoist on a mission. Their transport was killed and Larry had been struck in the ass when a well-aimed round came up through the floor.

They returned with the KIA, warning ahead that Larry had suffered a bad gut wound. He was pale and in shock. We were waiting for him at the landing pad. As soon as the chopper set down, in a chaotic rush, we pulled Larry out of its belly onto a stretcher and rushed him into Alpha Med, our make-shift clinic, in order to try and stabilize him for the longer trip to the Danang Naval Support Facility Hospital. We always cared for our own guys even more vigorously than usual, which was always full-tail boogey.

It really shook everyone to the core when a close buddy was wounded. We fought for each other. We knew about each other, hearing about our lives back home. We cared for each other. During the efforts to treat his injuries, Larry himself was in great spirits. He gave us a big smile and the thumbs-up signal.

"I made it, you guys. I just bought me a one-way ticket home. I'm goin' fishin' with the old man. Come visit us when you get home."

We hurried him into the rudimentary operating room. We were frantic. We knew Larry was bleeding badly. We had no option but to open him up and try to tie off the major bleeders. On site, we had no replacement blood, as we were painfully aware.

We discovered in surgery that the bullet had perforated his intestines, before exploding in his pancreas, which was shredded. His abdomen was a terrible mess. We knew he was a goner. That realization pierced us like the horn of a raging bull, but we had to push our own intense pain and anguish aside.

In denial that Larry was a goner, we tried desperately to somehow save him. We picked out shrapnel from his bowel and pancreas. We sewed up holes. We did everything we could and then shipped him to Danang, hanging on to a desperate and dwindling hope for the improbable miracle to occur.

I collapsed physically while my mental torment raged.

Why? Motherfuckers!

For four days, Larry lay in a hospital bed. At first, he exhibited pretty good spirits. He thought he'd made it. He thought he was going home. However, we knew better. His pancreas was leaking digestive enzymes into his abdominal cavity. By the second day he became swollen and bloated. There was nothing we could do. His shattered abdominal organs were shutting down. He screamed and hollered. Hallucinating, he would talk to his dad as if they were on a fishing trip. Then his eyes bulged out and he retched and heaved with little trickles of blood-tinged mucous dripping from the sides of his mouth. He was eating himself alive.

In his final days, Larry's skin had become thin and pale, his body bloated, and pinkish froth dribbled from his mouth. His delirium had gotten quieter, his fishing trips with his old man less frequent, his breathing shallow. That evening he died. All that remained of that strapping Okie kid with the shock of dirty blond hair was a bloated, pinkish-blue cadaver.

During the Vietnam war, approximately 10,000 USMC corpsmen served, many in hospital settings with others inserted into the battlefields. 645 were killed and 3,300 were wounded.

We'd just lost one of the best of them.

Distinguishing a Group of Fallen Vets with Seven Members

Besides Devil Docs and other brave corpsmen, we also lost physicians, though not many. During the Vietnam War, there were seven confirmed combat-related flight surgeon deaths: two in a 1966 fire on the USS Oriskany in the Gulf of Tonkin, one in a fixed wing crash, one in a rocket attack. And one of the three lost in helicopter crashes, was our own Lt. Curtis Baker. He was killed on March 28, 1967 when a chopper went down. He flew with VMO-2 MAG 16 in the UH-1E Huey and was my roommate at the Phu Bai base. He'd just relieved me there and I was headed to our Marble Mountain facility, when I heard about the fatal crash. Curt always joked about wearing white socks. When asked to identify his body, that's how I did it – by his white socks. I stayed with him, prior to his body being shipped out.

My buddies keep dying.

My mind – it is frying in agony, like an egg dropped into an over-heated pan.

Please.

Let me die.

To end this torment.

Losing Our Own to Pure Prideful Stupidity

At this stage in the war, we were meeting enemy forces that were better trained and equipped. They were punching, we were countering – both with increasing ferocity. Our commanders were aware that the NVA continued to re-supply its forces through what's known as the Ho Chi Minh Trail, a clandestine military supply route from North Vietnam through the mountains of Laos, Cambodia and South Vietnam, where massive amounts of weapons, ammunition and manpower were

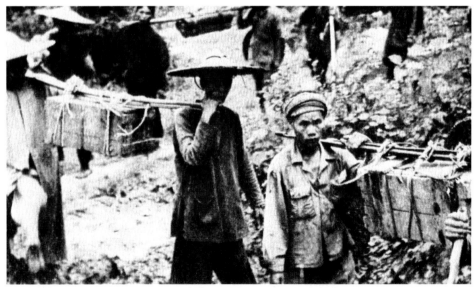

Viet Cong troops and local inhabitants transport guns and supplies along the Ho Chi Minh trail (Credit: U.S. Army)

being moved southward.

What we weren't fully aware of was how this heightened activity was in preparation for their surprise upcoming 1968 Tet Offensive, an all-out military campaign to be launched throughout South Vietnam simultaneously in multiple cities and regions.

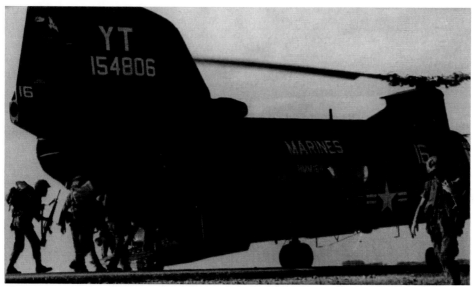

U.S. Marine Reconnaissance Team boards a CH-46 transport (Credit: USMC)

To gain intelligence on the movement of the enemy's soldiers, equipment and supplies, our commanders had designed Secret Reconnaissance Insert missions. In our CH-46A helicopters, we'd fly small teams of Army Special Forces and Marine Corps Force Reconnaissance troops to in their words, "secretly position them behind enemy lines."

Secretly?

Have you flown a helicopter in a combat zone?

They hear you coming.

They're waiting for you.

They'll ambush you.

Frequently, we'd get the urgent call from one of these brilliantly conceived missions.

"Emergency extract!"

We leapt into action, launching two CH-46As and two Huey gunships. We'd often have to fight our way in and out of a rescue mission.

137

After we'd lost a few dozen guys, the commanders decided to blame the casualties on an intelligence leak. They claimed to have plugged it and issued orders to continue their ill-conceived operations. Then, after losing yet another crew, we called a meeting in the operations shack.

"Intelligence leak, bullshit!"

One of the pilots, David Petteys, who had been involved in trying to drop these teams and instantly encountering enemy forces, writes "Khe Sanh is infested by at least three regiments of NVA. We can't put any reconnaissance teams out around the hillsides without them being immediately surrounded. We only have two battalions up there. So they're running nickel-dime company sweeps to clear out regiments! Are you kidding me? But oh, no, the Marines can hack it! After all, to call on the Army would be bad for the 'Marine Corps Reputation.' Thus, we slaughter the 19-year-olds so the Marine colonels and generals don't lose face at their cocktail parties."

At our meeting, one of our young reserve lieutenants grumbled, "Why doesn't the General come out here and listen to these roaring shitboxes? How do we get out of running these rotten missions?"

"How about mutiny?" chuckled another reservist.

"How about it?" came the question. "It sure as hell beats being dead".

Sorry We Be Crapping Our Pants

"I've got a better idea," I chimed in. "Why don't we all get diarrhea, and I'll ground the squadron."

"Yeah, that's a great idea!" was the roaring response.

"We all got diarrhea and the quack says we can't fly. We're grounded!"

Although it had been only a half-serious suggestion, word of it quickly got back to the Danang headquarters. This crazy flight quack was going to shut the squadron down if the mission wasn't scrapped. That was near-mutiny. To quash further trouble, Operations sent the message to halt all further secret recon inserts. Somehow, this news worked better than paregoric for clearing diarrhea, and our threat of revolt was instantly abated.

However, news of our mischief didn't create any levity among the brass.

We got a visit from General Krulak, "The Brute," Commander of Fleet Marine Force Pacific, who'd awarded me with my Bronze Star citation. He called us to the safety of the Danang Air Base for a visit to our squadron to hear him out.

"I just want you men to know that we are proud of you. You are real Marines. You have performed admirably and bravely under fire," and so on and so on. Then he lowered the boom. "And tomorrow morning we are going to restart the Secret Recon Inserts."

The guys looked at me. For an ordinary Marine, anyone who objected would be severely reprimanded. I was a doctor, already established in my career. They wanted me to speak out.

"Say something, Doc," Duffy whispered into my ear as he leaned slightly toward in an attempt not to catch the general's attention.

"General Krulak, sir." I offered, raising my hand.

"Yes, Doc?"

"Sir, don't you think the enemy can see and hear where we're going when we fly these big birds over the quiet jungle?" I asked. "And besides, we can pass over an entire enemy division without even knowing it," pointing out what I thought was obvious. "Why don't the recon guys walk in so the enemy can't see or hear them? Doesn't that make more sense?"

The general glared at me, turning a glorious beet red. "You have no military training. You're wrong, Doctor!" he shouted as he turned on his heels and stalked out of the room.

"Court-martial that man," was his exiting instruction to my commanding officer.

Please! Do It.

The next few days, the squadron buzzed.

Everyone wondered whether their quack would be court-martialed. I could only hope! That would mean I would have to trade my underground sand bagged bunker, plus my C-rations, and on top of that, my continuous combat exposures with the horrors of war for get this – clean sheets, three square meals a day, and an expedition through the military court system.

"Don't throw me in that briar patch, Br'er Krulak, please don't cast me down to have my gold buttons cut off!" I mimicked to whoever would listen.

Finally, the word came down: no court-martial. After all, I was one of their heroes. Ha! The truth was that if I got sent to the rear to be court-martialed, they'd have had to replace me. Nobody – but nobody – wanted to come up to the DMZ and take over for me.

In the American military, spit and polish, fancy salutes and big parades are the bailiwick of the regular officers. Heavy combat and dying are the responsibility of the reservists.

We are the expendables. Human expenditures in the hundreds of thousands. Husbands, fathers, sons and grandsons.

Bullet With Your Name

WHOP-WHOP-WHOP
"Medevac! Medevac!"
Me?
It was hot day. It had just rained again. It was tortuously humid. I'd finally gotten off to sleep, but once again I was needed for a mission.
Is today my day to die?
Because I was a little hungry, I figured it had to be around lunchtime.
Can't stop now!
Springing into action – laden with cement shirt, helmet, guns, Unit 1, and ass insurance, I sprinted through the sticky mud in a dead run toward the old UH-34D chopper that its co-pilot was firing up. The gunner was vaulting aboard, with the crew chief at a full gallop right ahead of me and the pilot not far behind. In only a few seconds after we'd clambered aboard, we were off, as I threw my ass insurance against the forward bulkhead and plopped down.
Replacements? I've asked, assholes!
To ease my tension, I tried to engage the gunner, Willy Arganza, a Chicano from Texas. Arganza was a wiry guy with olive skin and a swarthy complexion. Although Willy liked to act out the Frito Bandito, he was actually a bright, sensitive kid, quick to chime along with my

attempts at distracting ourselves with humor.

"Hey Willy, how come these damn grunts always get shot just when we're nodding off for a nice snooze?" I shouted over the din of the chopper.

"I don't know, Doc. There's always some cabron out there. I was in the middle of lunch when this call came in."

"Here comes the Doc," I shouted, "In this here bag I got a sure cure for acute lead poisoning."

"Hey, Doc," laughing, he screamed back, "I didn't know you carried tequila."

"Great idea, Willy! Tell the driver up front to stop at the next bar. Margaritas all around – on me!"

"Hey, Doc. We stop around here, we get our ass shot off. But that's okay, man. We got the quack aboard. We ain't losing nobody."

That comment disturbed me.

I was sitting there scared spitless because I knew we were all flawed, and nobody's invulnerable to a fatal dose of hot lead. As I sat back, periodically checking my equipment, time seemed suspended in the noisy draft of the chopper's belly. Momentarily, it will explode into frantic action. Who knows what we will encounter? My attention snapped back to Willy and the crew chief listening intently through the intercom, as they appeared to be getting word from the pilots.

"Hot zone! Hot zone, Doc!" The crew chief shouted.

Sitting squarely on my ass insurance, I crouched down while they manned their guns as we started a steep descent – a violent one eighty degree turn before hitting the ground. Through the door, a group of grimy grunts, heads down, carrying their wounded buddy on a litter, threw him aboard.

One of them leaned in and shouted to the crew chief, "How many can you carry?"

"How many you got?"

"We got two KIAs. Can you take 'em?"

"Bring'm!"

Quickly signaling with his colleagues, the grunts loaded two more litters with bodies covered completely with khaki ponchos, except for the boots. These guys' feet pointed in the same direction. They'd been dead for a while. Our wounded guy had an ABD pad on his gut. His eyes were open. He was breathing. He might make it.

The engine bellowed its mighty roar, and the chopper vibrated as it struggled to get airborne. As it skimmed along at treetop level trying to gain enough airspeed to begin the climb, both gunners opened up, enveloping the entire chopper belly in ear-shattering staccato reports and filling the air with the smell of gunpowder. The hot, spent shells rained over me as I crouched against the forward bulkhead covering my head with my arms.

Shortly, the mayhem ceased and we were airborne. I took my arms down and noticed they were wet, covered with blood. I looked over at the wounded man. His face was now ashen, his eyes glassy, his mouth ajar, his chest gouged wide open where a gaping exit wound had ripped through his chest and lungs. A round had come through the floor and driven chopper skin and floor matting through his body and sprayed us with blood and bits of tissue. I checked to see if Willy was hurt.

"I'm okay, Doc. What can you do for that guy?" Willy shouted as he gazed at his gory demise.

"He's gone, man. He's gone." I told him, trembling uncontrollably at the sight of blood pooling in the grunt's excavated chest. Willy looked at his own arms, trying to brush off the slimy flesh that had sprayed on his flight suit.

"Doc, I'm sick."

He puked, quickly turning away, trying to direct his vomit out the window. I would have joined him, but my gut was empty. My chest was as tight as a timber hitch. I wrenched nothing but gasping breaths.

Then I Saw His Wedding Ring

With the war's escalation, we were flying continuously, often multiple missions a day from the battlefields to the field hospitals. I became an automaton. I really stopped thinking and feeling. On the front lines, you never really rested. You ate little. You existed psychotically in a world apart.

WHOP-WHOP-WHOP!

Shit! I'd think immediately. But instantaneously, as the call for me came, I would break into a dead run.

Where's the corpsman?

There's nobody else, fool!

Taking off this time, all I knew was it was a real emergency, but that was all. No one could tell me exactly what happened, but it sounded like a gut wound. Those were some of the worst. The poor grunt who is split or blown open around his abdomen, he's spewing blood, fecal matter and urine all over you. Trying to evaluate a wound like this under these extreme circumstances is like digging in a filthy, opaque pool of blood, flesh and dirt, looking for what was cut or torn and bleeding. These are real emergencies and my mind raced as I collected my gear, throwing in four or five bottles of albumin.

This guy's gonna need this real bad.

I also snatched my helmet, cement shirt, flak jacket, and ass insurance. Laden with my 30 pounds of equipment, as was now unmercifully routine, I sprinted out of the hootch door in a frantic dash to the shuddering bird about a hundred yards away.

This heat's oppressive!

It's like being slow baked in an oven.

I can barely breathe.

The air is choking me.

All this crap we're constantly breathing in.

If we don't die today, we will in a few decades.

Making matters just that much more unbearable, it had just rained again. I ran in ground so soggy, I'd sink in my boots to my ankles in the thick red mud. Soaking wet, my filthy feet gave off their own quite distinctive odor – a mixture of aviation fuel and ripe body odor.

Somehow, my body ignored my brain which was screaming about being too fatigued. That cruel internal conflict must be what the characters felt in Dante's Inferno, while carried along. However, this was reality.

Our hell was real, living and breathing its fire upon us.

Once this mission was airborne, flying over patches of lush jungle, my mind pondered how I just couldn't get accustomed to such natural beauty, being subjected to the destructiveness of warfare and the obliteration of a world once so serene.

All of a sudden I started rolling around in the helicopter. Our pilot was doing some fancy dancing to get down into the landing zone, making diversionary moves to keep the gooks on the ground guessing as to exactly where we were going to drop in.

Must be enemy action down there.

Then we really plummeted earthward and hit the ground.

Around our landing zone, the grunts had formed a perimeter. Four ran to the chopper with this guy on a stretcher. Tied to his belly I spotted an ABD pad – a thick twelve-by-twelve gauze used to cover large abdominal wounds. He was unconscious but breathing.

This guy was a grubby one, with a week's growth of stubble on his face, his whole body caked with mud, sweat and piss – which had liquefied in his armpits and crotch. He reeked of rancid sweat and dry urine. This crud was grubbier than the worst stumblebum I'd seen back in Chicago's Cook County Hospital. I wouldn't want to even touch them. His comrades threw this dude like a sack of potatoes onto the chopper's floor. Rushing to get airborne, we had to get the hell out of there as fast as we possibly could because we knew the gooks were coming after us.

Seeing this heap of shit up close for the first time, I noticed that his beard was matted, his mouth foul, dry and parched, his face covered with infected mosquito bites as he gasped for breath. He was ashen gray, like a gritty old alcoholic overdosed on rotgut. I found it hard to believe this nasty human was somebody's kid, but as I began to look him over, I spotted something shiny and clean on his left hand, something that didn't fit with this gritty, foul body – a gold band on the fourth finger of his left hand.

It was his wedding ring.

It looked like the only thing this guy kept clean, all that he really cared about. That sudden awareness thumped my head hard and re-ignited my soul. This kid was married! This poor, cruddy bastard was a newlywed! He'd surely looked different at his wedding, all clean-shaven and smiling with bright eyes and pink cheeks. He must have been the pride of his parents, his family and all of friends.

This sure ain't a John Wayne movie.

Glamorous.

Glorious.

Bull shit!

Oh well, to hell with it.

Right now, I've got a job to do.

As this his kid's wretched body lay stretched out on the floor of the chopper, vibrating in harmony with this smelly flying contraption, I started looking for a vein to start IV albumin, anticipating his blood pressure could drop out. As I felt his arm, I noticed my hand was hot, sticky and wet. Fresh warm blood was oozing from around the ABD pad.

Hope I don't have to open up that pack.

Damn it!

All of that could really come spilling out all over me.

At first, I tried to leave it. Then, I noticed more blood. Soon, there was much more blood. This poor guy was bleeding out through his abdomen. I had no choice but to go in there to see what I could do about stopping the massive hemorrhaging. Gingerly, I began to lift the ABD pad from his belly. As I lifted, the blood began gushing out. I ripped off the pad to find a gaping hole in his gut. His small intestines were bulging out of it.

Oh Jesus... How do I stop this?

From my Unit 1, I grabbed for the hemostats. How the hell was I going to find the freaking bleeder? We didn't have any lights in this shithouse. Besides, it was vibrating like a washing machine's spin cycle. The hemostats were designed to stop bleeders, carefully placed in a controlled operating room. Here? I'd never be able to even find the bleeder. I only had one option, as I hurriedly concluded – the hole was big enough to allow my right hand through into it. I'd just feel around to see if I could find the bleeder. I caught myself. My hands were filthy, I hadn't washed them in days, so how the hell could I stick these filthy paws into this abdomen? Because I had no other chance – or he was going to bleed out!

Goddamn, I've gotta to do something!

Must do this!

By then, blood began forming a pool on the chopper's floor. It was all over me. The crew chief and gunner just sat watching me. They didn't know what to do. They watched, helpless, as I poked around with my hand in the abdomen, where I felt the aorta throbbing, then a stream of hot liquid flowing, surging against the palm of my hand in time with the heartbeats.

Okay, I've got a hold of the renal artery.

I grabbed the broken artery, to close it off between my thumb and forefinger as I felt the aorta surge with each heartbeat. His pulse was really getting fast. I had to stop the hemorrhaging.

"I've got to stop the damn bleeding!" I shouted to the anxious crew.

Somehow I accomplished that as the blood had stopped gushing but continued to ooze. If I could hold onto that bleeder, maybe we could save him in the operating room when we got down on the ground. His pulse must have been one twenty now but getting thready. We were losing him – threadier and weaker, threadier and weaker. What an unreal feeling to have your hand in some guy's stomach, feeling him die – feeling him die in my own hands, and I had failed to prevent it.

"Damn it to hell, you rotten asshole! Stop bleeding! Please, stop."

At this point, I was weeping, begging, and screaming at this soon-to-be corpse, my flight suit covered with blood, my right arm completely drenched up to the elbow, the floor awash with blood clots. The kid gasped, his face almost white. His heart gave out a few final feeble thrusts.

He was gone and I was nauseated. I felt the urge to vomit. I got the dry heaves and started retching and heaving as I pulled my hand out of the hot, wet hole in his abdomen. I covered it up with the soggy ABD pad, wiped my hands on my flight suit, and huddled down for the rest of the ride. I had tears and vomit streaming down my face. I was crying and retching all at once. What an ignominious way to die. That had been somebody's loved one – reduced to filthy and vile-smelling rubbish.

God bless *America! God* damn *America!*

Jump In With Us Porky Bastards

If only I could replace this dead kid with one of those war profiteers, or some slimy politician, or a lardy labor leader. They'd be lying here in this vibrating privy with their guts hanging out, instead of this young husband with a future.

Right now, a wife, a mother and father don't know what I do. But soon, they will. I'd seen what happened. I'm glad they are free of those memories. I will never be.

How they must have worried and prayed for him. For his safe return home.

So horribly needless.

A soldier, lay on a litter,
Rigid, immobile,
In the shock-ice,
Of fear and pain,
Into twilight sleep,
Falling,
Never to see the care in her smile,
Or hear the sanity of her jokes,
Falling,
Never to feel the touch,
That wiped Asian dust from his forehead.
Kathie Swazuk
Vietnam Combat Nurse

Finally Driven Completely Crazy

While the senseless carnage fueled my rage, when one of my close comrades burned to death in a chopper crash, I went genuinely insane. His name was Captain J.A. "Jack" House, an HMM 265 Dragons pilot of true valor with a passion for aviation. We'd compete fiercely at acey-ducey. We spoke of flying and family. He adored Amy, his beautiful wife and the love of his life. He talked endlessly about being a new father. Just prior to his final mission, Jack had been exuding excitement about an upcoming R&R where he was going to see his baby boy.

On June 30, 1967, fresh off of the grueling Battle for Khe Sanh, Jack was flying an

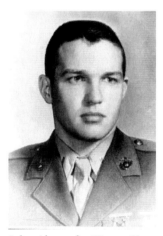

John Alexander House, II
Captain
HMM-265, MAG-16, 1ST
MAW, III MAF
USMC

11-man reconnaissance team into a drop zone inside a heavily protected enemy stronghold when his aircraft was hit with small arms, automatic weapons and anti-aircraft fire. It burst into flames. He managed to fly the disabled bird for a short distance before it crashed.

I was flying a routine transport in the area when we heard the mayday call. We were minutes away. Dropping into the LZ, I jumped out and dashed to the flaming wreckage. I saw Jack trapped in the cockpit, burned to death. And then I smelled the fetid odor. My gut twisted. I began to retch.

We were under intense enemy fire at the time. I saw no one else alive, just a few dead bodies on the ground. I fled back to our chopper and we got out safely.

Shit. Why me?

Why did I have to see this?

I will relive this every day of my life.

I will never escape it.

Only if I die.

Mistaken Killing by 'Friendly Military Action'

Flying over Vietnam, away from the cities, you see the rural landscape, dotted with clusters of communities, surrounded by well-kept agricultural fields. Northwest of Khe Sanh, a small village called Lang Vei was populated primarily by Montagnards, a race made up of various indigenous ethic groups, whose name means mountain dwellers. Commonly, they were known as highlanders, a dwarf-like aboriginal people with a primitive culture, who existed in a more or less autonomous state. During the war, they were fierce fighters, recruited heavily by the ARVN (Army of the Republic of Vietnam) as mercenaries in the U.S. backed military operations, particularly with our Special Forces.

This majestic landscape and these ancient villages were deeply impacted by bombings and herbicides as we attempted to shut down the Ho Chi Minh Trail. During the war, overrun by Viet Cong forces, it's been estimated that over 200,000 Montagnards died and 85% of their communities were destroyed.

Tragically, we were responsible for one of them.

"This is what the war ended up being about: we would find a VC

village, we called for jets, sweeping down and screaming, first drop-
ping bombs that blew the rubble and debris to ashes, then napalm that
burned ashes to nothing. Then the village was not a village."

Bryan Alec Floyd
The Long War Dead

In the fall of 1967, two Air Force F-4s returning from a raid on North Vietnam apparently had not discharged their full loads of bombs. Landing an airplane with live munitions aboard constitutes such a difficult and dangerous maneuver that pilots are required to first discharge any remaining load. In this instance, they decided to identify a target of opportunity upon which to do that. Being so close to the DMZ and with dusk obscuring adequate visualization of land-marks, the pilots mistook Lang Vei for a North Vietnamese village.

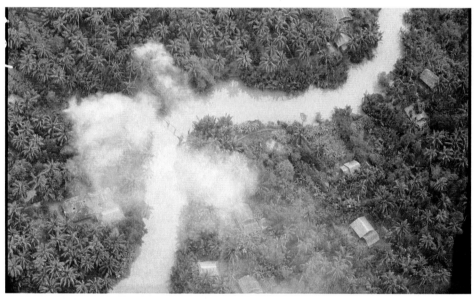

Aerial of U.S. bombing of Vietnamese village (Credit: National Archives)

We were told that the attack had taken only about five minutes but managed to level the hamlet completely and kill forty to forty-five of its residents. In an attempt to salvage as many of the wounded as possible, the Marines from Khe Sanh dispatched their general medi-cal officer and a group of medical corpsmen. Since this U.S. military outpost had an airstrip at which KC-130s could land, they used these large twin-engine fixed-wing cargo planes to Medevac the more se-verely wounded. Our squadron was therefore not called in to provide support for any of those operations. Nevertheless, the morning after the incident, we went to Lang Vei to help out.

Only a few thatched-roof huts remained standing. Most of homes still smoldered from the fires of twelve hours earlier. We were the first to arrive to access the aftermath. We searched the area for the dead or any possible remaining wounded trapped in the smoky debris. In order to cover maximal territory in minimal time, we split up and walked through, about twenty feet abreast, identifying fatalities and listening for cries.

Charley called out to Matt, "I got one here."

I hollered over to Charley, "Is he alive?"

Charley answered, "It's a woman." His voice shaking, "Her head's crushed. She's been dead for a while."

I kept on walking and came upon the rubble of a charred hut. I peered inside.

Did I just see something moving?

Among the lifeless bodies, I noticed an infant that must not have been more than two months old, charred black, but alive. I saw his tiny lips opening and closing in a deep sucking reflex. His stiff and rigid body had been burned beyond repair.

With that surge of nausea I'd come to know as my shadow whenever I encountered one of the great horrors of my Vietnam experience, my first impulse was to call out. Then I decided not to. My second impulse was to attempt to pick the child up. I rejected that because I realized that if I did that, his limbs may fall off or his skin crack open, exposing his innards.

This baby is dying.

I am a goddamn pediatrician... but absolutely powerless.

I wanted to just turn away and leave it as it was, hoping soon his suffering would end. But I couldn't stop staring at his innocent puckers. I couldn't leave him, and I couldn't take him either.

A terrible sense of impotence welled up in me. It was a response I'd come to know only too well, one that repeatedly arose on Medevac missions, because they brought me guys barely alive and asked me to save them. Just like this child, our boys are in hopeless shape, and I'm prying around under bloody ponchos, without any information from anybody about what is wrong with them. Light is poor and steadiness of movement impossible, swaying like a palm tree in stormy winds. Even when I could find out what was going on, that thin strand tying my patient to life was unraveling and there was nothing I could do – except feel gut-wrenching despair.

There I was again in the presence of a pitiful end to an innocent life. What could I do to mercifully end the suffering now that mortal harm had been done? What should I do? Slowly, I removed my .38 special from its holster, held its muzzle three inches from that tiny, blackened forehead, and pulled the trigger.

At that moment, part of me also perished.

Chancy called over, "Hey, Doc, what are you doing'?"

"Nothing. Chancy. Nothing. Don't worry about it." I pulled some flooring debris over the baby's now lifeless body so he wouldn't be exposed and walked off, so pitifully sad, sickened and enraged by what I had to do.

It went fast.

It didn't hurt, I hope.

Uncle Sam – you killed him.

Me?

I am your finger on the trigger.

Chapter Eight
Moments of Respite

"Happy hour with alcohol was a means to dilute the days of boredom and to temporarily erase the moments of screaming sounds of human agony, to wash away the residual visions of the pieces of flesh torn apart—the hidden truths of real war."
H. Lee Bell
1969

We got time off – in the rears, so to speak. In fact, we'd either be in the thick of fighting trying to say alive or dying of boredom. Down time was called not only R&R but I&I, which stands for intoxication and intercourse. Actually, I stayed mostly sober and totally chaste – a loyal married man. But, as Marines, especially combat soldiers, we needed escapes from our forbidding duties.

Our enemy was active day and night. And we were chronically short-handed – guys were getting killed or going home. Consequently, time off was enthusiastically well-received.

We loved hearing updates about fresh replacements arriving. We hooted with excitement while exhaling a comforting sigh of relief.

I am still alive, folks.

Food, Hot Water and Clean Clothes

When there's calm, you think about food, hot soapy water and clean clothes. In combat, personal hygiene is a joke. You pee and crap in a hole. You eat, on occasion. Between bombings, you catch a few winks of nervous slumber. So, when those moments of respite arrive, first you find a real bathroom and then chow down. It's really a big deal just being able to piss and shit somewhere other than your pants. In battle, you stop to do either, you might die. You've basically lived in your flight suit. To disrobe, you'd peel it off of your body that reeked of decaying flesh, which is exactly what it was.

153

You always did what you could for your feet. In combat, they take a hell of a beating. You need them, though, to survive. Leave your boots on too long, you develop what's called immersion foot, recognizable when your skin peels off in your socks.

On one occasion, as I lay on my cot, waiting to take off on leave, the door smashed open and the sunny voice of my replacement, Art Lochridge, hollered, "Levin, get your fuckin' ass out of here, you lazy bastard. They need you now in Danang at the O Club."

"Well, shit, sir," I retorted, "Do you mean to tell me they're overloaded on San Miguel beer?" I hugged him and after we shook hands warned him, "Art, it's really bad out there. Watch your ass and try not to fly Medevacs."

"I will, Al. Why don't you just get out of here and rest up?"

Moments of Tranquility from the Storm

That day, the flight to Danang proved exceptionally glorious. As usual, the pilots flew at about five thousand feet over the ocean about a mile or so from the shore to minimize exposure to ground fire. Although we always had to be vigilant for possible small arms fire, it was unlikely that anything that could cause major damage would come from that area.

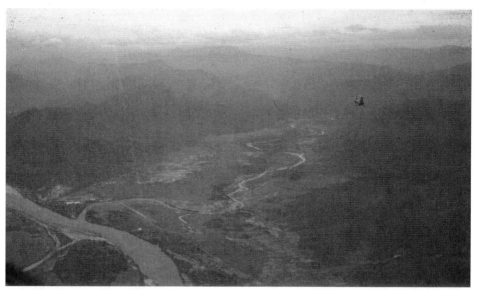

Aerial of northern South Vietnam's mountainous landscape with helicopters in flight (Credit: Wikimedia Commons)

On this particular route, we felt relatively secure.

That's what I love about flying: every time you look down to the ground, everything looks clean and well-ordered. With the rhythmic vibrations and the overpowering roar of the engines, the whop of the rotors, and the rush of air streaming by the chopper, it generates a unique feeling of freedom from any constraints. Flying through quiet skies, I could sink into an introspective, relaxed state, transfixed by the beauty of the jungle, the ocean and seashore.

All too soon, however, I began to see the familiar signs that indicated Marble Mountain lay ahead – Red Beach with its radio facilities, then Monkey Mountains and the gun emplacements. Soon we started descending. The loud roar of the engines shifted, the rotor blades shuddered, and then the main mounts thudded onto the landing strip, where as always we first taxied toward the fuel pits. The gunner and crew chief jumped out, pulled the fuel nozzles, and refueled the bird while it was running. We then taxied into the bird's revetment, an area on the landing field bounded on three sides by sandbags to protect the choppers from artillery and mortar fire, also reducing battle damage that attacks could cause to the field.

As the pilot shut the bird down, I gathered my gear – my M-14, my revolver, my Unit 1, my duffel bag in which I'd stored the remnants of a blood-and-vomit-stained flight suit, some dirty underwear, and a filthy, stinking sleeping bag. After jumping from the chopper, I unconsciously patted my waistline to reaffirm the presence of the belt holding my .38 special and my trusty survival knife. In the hot and muggy air, I pulled off my flight helmet and threw it in the bag, pulled out a wrinkled, dusty fatigue cap and donned it while starting the long quarter-mile walk to my hootch.

As I walked alone, too bone tired to think about the recent events, I began to plan my ritual. I would go through my "Wow, I'm still alive!" rites. Then, I would begin to address the fact that I smelled like I was dead. I'd head for a shit, shower, shave and shampoo.

God, to feel human again.

Ignoring Injury and Pain

On this occasion, while enjoying the glorious experience of cleaning up, I was all alone. It was the middle of the afternoon and no one was around. For a few minutes I had sat on one of the benches anticipating the sensual joy of hot water on my tortured body. Then I stood up and with the movements of a sleazy stripteaser began to slowly remove my seedy flight suit. I unzipped from mid-chest to down beyond my crotch, then pulled the suit from my left shoulder and let it droop down the middle of my arm as I removed it from my right shoulder and slowly wriggled out of it, watching it drop past my waist to down around my knees.

Then I saw it. Then it hit me. My entire right hip displayed a mass of purple and green hematoma. It was resolving. In fact, the greenish area indicated that it had been there for a while. A few days earlier, we were shot down during a mission and I'd hit my right hip on an ammo box, while making a crash landing. Now, that I finally noticed it, I shrieked in pain and collapsed onto the floor, where I lay crying hysterically and pounding the boards.

All of a sudden the pain that I'd ignored had become almost unbearable. I couldn't walk. I couldn't stand up. Then a horrible realization struck me. This had happened five days ago, and I had completely blotted it out. I had completely disregarded it.

God, I hurt. So badly.

Without pain, you can lose one of nature's most critical clues that enough is enough. Anyone who shuts it out is on the road to self-destruction. By completely disregarding my own self-preservation, the realization struck me that even the primitive will to survive had left me. Now, I sensed that if I made it out of Vietnam alive, it wouldn't be by my own doing, but just random chance. That truly frightened me. Without pain, without the clues of nature, you can easily go on and destroy yourself without ever knowing you've done it.

After lying on the floor for nearly an hour, I decided it was ridiculous to lie around any longer, stupid to feel sorry for myself. If I was going to die, I was going to die and that was all there was to it.

Damn it, Levin, stop sniveling.

Get going.

Fortunately, the pain from my injury lessened substantially. I was able to regain my mobility, finish undressing, shower and shave, dowsing myself with deodorant and after-shave. Then I left the shower building with a towel around my waist, carrying all of my toiletries and soiled clothes. I knew I couldn't just continue ignoring my injury.

Back in the hootch, I donned a clean fatigue uniform and went over to the dispensary, where I showed my hip to Kurt Bohiman, a general medical officer. Upon examination, X-rays revealed small areas of calcification around the soft tissue injury and a hairline fracture of the greater trochanter of the right femur. Because it was a non-weight-bearing bone, I'd been able to run and carry heavy loads.

After I described how it happened, we put it in the record, so that in the future, if arthritis developed in that joint, at least some pencil pusher in military benefits couldn't accuse me of being a faker.

A fucker, maybe, but certainly not a faker.

Gorging on My Chile Con Carne

On the endless boring nights when we were inactive, we would all gather around to talk about women, fine food and booze. One evening I started bragging, describing to the fellows how I had been a cook at Delta Gamma Sorority. There, I assured them, I learned to prepare the world's greatest chili – what the girls all called my Celestially Endowed Chili. It was a bowlful of heavenly satisfaction.

"Gentlemen, let me tell you about how I learned to make chili. It was a dark and stormy night and I was lying in my bed trying to sleep when the lightning and thunder jolted me awake. Then, all of a sudden, from a dark cloud overhead came a bolt of shiny lightning, then a golden beam that transformed into a golden staircase. Down that staircase came an ancient man with a long white beard carrying a pair of tablets. I squinted. I looked hard. I wondered why he was coming toward me, and then, as he came closer, I could see that on the tablets was written a recipe for chili con carne." Needless to say, this story created a fanfare of hoots and hollers and applause. After that I regaled them with the accolades of my concoction. "Once the Pope called me because he wanted to use it for Holy Water, but it was too messy. Ya' know, his white clothes and all."

After all the braggadocious chatter about my meaty delight and how it made the sorority sisters swoon, the guys forced me to put my money – or more precisely, my cooking – where my mouth was. Jack, one of our senior pilots, got up and said, "Okay, Doc, you think you're such a good chili maker, then make us some fucking great chili, Chef Boy R Delicioso." At that moment, the gauntlet had been dropped. I had been challenged. I was, therefore, morally obliged to replicate my world-renowned culinary masterpiece.

But I decided not to bring it on until the squadron would be able to enjoy the essence of my creation without any rude interruptions. So, I waited until combat action waned, because right at that time, reasonably regular artillery attacks forced us to sleep in our bunkers – those holes in the ground that we shared with lice, rats, and a variety of other creepy and crawling creatures.

Finally, that day came. Operations had slackened enough to allow me to put my chili where their mouths were. So, I went to the cook to see what we had, in order to put together whatever likely ingredients we could turn up – B-ration beef, beans, salt and pepper, Tabasco, Worcestershire, and lots of Louisiana hot sauce. Brewing these odds and ends in a giant cauldron took almost half a day. As the odors wafted across the compound, I had many visits from my colleagues, who sampled the heavenly mixture's progress. I'm sure this chili didn't match anything that could've been made by a civilian in a real kitchen with the appropriate ingredients – to us, however, it was ambrosia.

That night, the whole squadron slopped down my Celestially Endowed Chili. Since it was the spiciest thing around, it was a great success. Everybody had three or four helpings, which made me feel extremely proud and vindicated. Everybody complimented me and told me that, indeed, I'd been correct in saying my chili was celestially endowed. Later still that night, however, we were explosively entertained by a major gastric visitation from the wrathful gods of the kitchen.

All of us began to fart uncontrollably. The epidemic of farting made me fearful that if someone stayed in his bunker we'd have a case of spontaneous combustion and the guy would blow himself up. On the other hand, if we'd slept on the top of our bunkers and had an artillery attack, we'd be killed. That entire night I fretted, worrying that either someone would asphyxiate in his bunker or get blown away sleeping on top. Surely, this was the first time in history that an entire squadron of United States Marines found itself placed in mortal jeopardy by such friendly fire.

Visiting Shelly

My dearest of friends Shelly was smart.

Like me, my old college friend and roommate had completed medical school on scholarships and odd jobs. To help pay for his education, Shelly joined the U.S. Army. As a regular officer, he was well cared for. He did his internship at Letterman Hospital in San Francisco. When he was shipped to Vietnam, he was assigned to Vung Tau, an R&R center for American and Vietnamese soldiers. As we were in Vietnam during the same year, I invited him to my duty station at the DMZ and was hurt when he declined my proffered hospitality. However, he invited me to Vung Tau, and I accepted. By then I was already insane.

I still wonder who in my shoes wouldn't have been.

I hitched a ride to Saigon on a C-130 loaded with KIAs that I had processed the night before. With me I carried my M-14, my survival knife, my .38 and a bandolier of 7mm ammunition. When we reached Saigon, I hitched a ride in a Huey loaded with repaired radio equipment. As we landed at Vung Tau, Shelly came running to the chopper to greet me. He had brought several friends with him. What I saw when I looked around was wall-to-wall gooks, crawling all over the place. There was no way I'd give up my arsenal. Shelly hollered, "Al, put down your guns! This is a non-combat zone."

"Says who, asshole?" I shouted over the engine's roar.

"Says the General. This is an R&R resort," Shelly implored.

"R&R my ass! These are gooks and this is war!"

"Well, at least put them down until we get to the barracks," he pleaded.

"Okay, schmuck, I'll trust you, but this is fuckin' scary."

Acting Crazy – Well, I Was

We walked from the air strip to the barracks about two hundred yards away. The compound looked like a college campus. After we reached where I would bunk, Shelly and his two friends, both general medical officers at the facility, pleaded with me to leave my weapons there. Finally, we struck a compromise. I would leave my rifle and ammunition in the barracks but would stuff my .38 into my baggy flight suit so that no one would see it. After that, we went out to do the town for a couple of days.

To this day, Shelly describes that visit as me looking and acting completely insane.

I was thin as a rail and wound as tight as a coiled snake – and probably, venomous.

I stared at everyone and constantly watched over my shoulder. Although I was totally unaware of anything amiss in my conduct then, Shelly assures me now that my crazy behavior really embarrassed him.

Special Landing Force Accommodations

By October of 1967, our squadron had been stretched out along the DMZ, between Dong Ha and Khe Sanh for months. We had engaged in the heaviest combat around that area at the time. We suffered many casualties. We cared for hundreds of wounded soldiers. We were depleted completely.

Due to our extreme fatigue, we were rotated onto the Special Landing Force – the SLF – an aircraft carrier battle group specially outfitted to handle helicopters and a battalion of infantry. Support for the SLF consisted of a task force that included light artillery and tanks. It was supposed to involve itself in "vertical assault" – dropping in on the enemy and attacking by surprise – quickly engaging them and relieving any pressure on beleaguered ground troops.

We used it for support or replacement, a sort of floating relief station. Instead of having to live in holes and eat C-rations, soldiers and airmen would live aboard ship with three cooked meals a day, sleep on clean sheets at night, and enjoy running water and plumbing for a significant period of time. Combat occurred only in the daytime. At night we slept safely away from any live action.

For us, SLF was a welcome break from bedlam and death. We always looked forward to that rotation. In addition to the advantages of shipboard living, when the Navy ship required refueling and mechanical repairs, as well as resupplying food and water, most Marine units on board went along and took liberty in the Philippines.

When our outfit came aboard, the Navy crew had been "at sea" for fifty-five days. I began to hear rumors that the ship was going to

Subic Bay to refit but commanders planned to offload our squadron onto the mainland. Enemy activity had intensified and they might need us while the ship was gone for ten days. Such a prospect angered me greatly. I knew we needed time off and I started politicking to keep us there. I went to the colonel to emphasize that we suffered from severe combat fatigue. We needed this chance for a few days' relaxation.

As our outfit's medical officer, I argued that we'd do better to take these ten days off, or we'd lose the efficiency of the entire squadron.

"We need not lose pilots from exhaustion," I warned.

I don't know whether the colonel believed me or whether he felt I would make too big a stink if they didn't let us go, but whatever the reason, they allowed our squadron to go along.

Pecker Rot

As a flight surgeon, one of my obligations now involved making sure our boys did not contract any venereal diseases while on R&R at Olongapo. This was a suburb of the large Navy base at Subic Bay, populated primarily by prostitutes whose activities the Philippine government controlled.

In those days, when penicillin-resistant gonococci were just emerging as a problem that we in the States had become aware of, these prostitutes were getting regular check-ups and penicillin injections – needed or not.

That didn't warrant carelessness.

I therefore made it my duty to give mandatory V.D. lectures to all of the approximately two thousand Marines on board the carrier. In the two days of transit between Vietnam and the Philippines, I gave no fewer than seventeen V.D. lectures in a large hangar bay. Attendance was required. My audiovisual equipment consisted of a microphone, a broomstick, and a bag of condoms.

"Gentlemen, it's called Pecker Rot. How do you avoid it? You don't fuck!"

At each and every one of my seventeen lectures, this advice always brought loud boos, accompanied by the shaking of fists and shouting from the audience as several grunts acted as if they were heading for the doors.

I did what I could to warn them. Still, the medical clinics still got flooded with patients in the days that followed.

Second Honeymoon

During my tour of duty in Vietnam, twice, I was granted expense-paid leave to visit my wife. I'd catch a transport to Okinawa and then a commercial airliner to Hawaii. What I only really remember from those occasions is that we copulated like a couple of rabbits.

Chapter Nine
War Is Profitable

New York Times Headline
Economy: 1966 Best Year, Says President
"Barring a sudden end of hostilities in Vietnam, 1967 will be
as good a year for business as 1966."
Gardner Ackley
President LBJ's Chief Economic Adviser

"I spent most of my time being a muscle-man for Big Business, Wall Street
and the Bankers. I was a racketeer, a gangster for capitalism."
USMC Major General Smedley D. Butler
War is a Racket
1935

When America went to war in Vietnam, it opened its public coffers. Over the 10+ year conflict, in today's money, we spent about a trillion dollars. Hundreds of billions went for war operations – personnel, weaponry, equipment and supplies. Billions more was poured into infrastructure to build airports, bases and medical care facilities. Some of LBJ's buddies at Brown and Root, a subsidiary of Halliburton, were known as the Vietnam builders. With America's pacification efforts in-country faltering, LBJ chose to dramatically escalate our military operations. Basically, we'd decided to bomb, shoot, poison or starve our enemies out of existence.

In the year I was there, the "Free World Forces" in Vietnam, comprised of Americans, Vietnamese, Koreans, Australians, Thais and Filipinos, reached a combined total of 1.3 million military personnel. That is one soldier for every fifteen South Vietnamese. With all of the intense fighting, the kill ratio was always in our favor, but we had gained nothing – neither control of territory or any reduction in the enemy's effectiveness.

Promising to end the war, Nixon got elected, but couldn't afford the political repercussions of losing it. The centerpiece of his policy was "Vietnamization," which entailed the build-up of the South Vietnamese armed forces and the draw-down of U.S. troops. This was the same strategy used earlier by the French, when its war in Indochina proved to be too expensive and politically divisive.

With our additional billions in financial resources, the GVN (Government of the Republic of Vietnam) drafted about half of the able-bodied male population in the country, many of whom were teenagers. By the end of 1970, the GVN had conscripted about 400,000 soldiers, for a total of 1.1 million. We also trained and generously armed them. With our support, for the first time, their infantry forces were supplied with M-16 rifles, grenade launchers and machine guns, the same we used. We imported helicopters, patrol boats, tanks, artillery, air transports and squadrons of F-5 tactical bombers.

Getting out proved to be even more costly than what we'd expended to conduct war operations. Our losses were immeasurable in terms of casualties. We also lost a lot of expensive military weaponry – approximately 10,000 aircraft – 3,744 planes, mostly F4 fighters at $2.4 million apiece, 5,607 helicopters were downed, with each Huey UH-1 costing almost a million dollars, and 578 Unmanned Aerial Vehicles were also destroyed. In terms of munitions, over 7 million tons of bombs were dropped, three and a half times more than WWII, or about a thousand pounds for every man, woman and child in the country.

Yet, even with our superior technology and firepower, we faced an enemy of guerilla-style fighters who battled the Chinese for a thousand years, then the French, then the Japanese and now the Americans.

As JFK's advisors had warned – the communists were able to appeal to the force of nationalism against the "white faces" with guns. America battled an enemy that was determined and ingenious. Our increased aggression only strengthened the resolve of the Vietnamese who were culturally inured to adversity and hardship. Our enemy shared a simple rallying cry from Ho Chi Minh: "We must sacrifice down to the last drop of our blood to defend our land."

An Institute for Defense Analysis report confirmed that, as of October of 1967, U.S. bombing of North Vietnam still had not reduced the flow of men and supplies to the south nor "weakened the determi-

nation of the North Vietnamese leaders to continue to directly support
he insurgency in the south."

But, fighting such a war generated huge profits for the defense industry and bulging political coffers. Is that why we were there? Among
the troops in the war, we had a saying: "They don't want us to win this
war. It's the only one they've got." We laughed, but really, we were just
covering our seething anger and pervading disillusionment.

Among the Snuffys, as they'd called the lower ranking soldiers
– the grunts thrown into the intense CQC (Close Quarters Combat)
fighting – the growing consensus was that lives were being wasted in a
proxy war with substandard weaponry while the higher-ranking military officers were focused on their careers and the fat cats were lining
their pockets.

The bottom line was the bottom line. Other than that, nobody
cared.

Flying Flash Bulbs

WHOSH-WHOSH-WHOSH!

Roaring like a dozen old fire engines in a deafening din, the
Sikorsky UH-34D helicopter came to life, as the big four-bladed rotor
of the bird spun up to speed. While my body acted in mindless auto-
mation running full speed towards this aircraft, I was fully aware of
this rust bucket I was boarding for the mission.

How do our boys keep this antique in the air?

This behemoth won't get shot down.

We'll crash on our own.

*We get two wounded grunts in this bird on a hot day... it'll strain
so hard... it'll collapse trying to lift itself into the air.*

Noticing our Huey gunships circling above, normally along to
protect us...

We need more of those, not these shuttering shithouses.

The Marines are too goddamn cheap.

*At least those behemoths can keep the gooks off our backs in case
we crash.*

Aboard our chopper for this mission were Casey, the pilot, Whit-
ey the co-pilot, Stubby the crew chief and Terry, our gunner. Inside

the belly of these ancient Medevac helicopters, there was always that rotten nauseating odor that permeates the air.

I stunk too. I was covered with dried blood from a poor bastard who'd bled out on me the day before. Clots of blood remained in my boots and on what was left of my socks. I was too tired to notice any of it, until now.

What never escapes you either are the searing fears that overtake you each time you're heading out. They rage even stronger hearing the call squawking "Emergency!" You know then you may drop in right into the middle of mind-numbing havoc. In the ensuing chaos, that terror, though, can somehow be converted to fuel superhuman tenacity, persistence and resolve.

Goddamn!

I'm scared out of my mind!

My mouth's as dry as paper.

I'm fuckin' starving.

Hell, we might end up barbecue.

Suddenly, our chopper lurched to the right and started coming down fast. Its engines continued to roar away. The blades vibrated violently, like a giant egg-beater. My body shook.

I'm absolutely terrified!

My heart pounded. My teeth vibrated. My chest heaved as I began hyperventilating. I was nauseated but did not vomit because I hadn't eaten anything.

My gut is frozen.

Then, the chopper hit the ground. To relieve stress, I started screaming dark humor at the top of my lungs.

"Damn it, Casey, you'd get fired from the airlines with crappy landings like that. Your passengers be screaming."

No one heard my senseless ramblings.

"Have a little compassion for my ass. You're sitting on a goddamn seat cushion, I'm on a fucking boiler plate."

As the engines went to idle with the blades still spinning, everybody in the belly sprang into action – Terry was up, poised, glaring out of the windows, sweeping the muzzle of his M-60 from fore to aft looking for gooks.

If that guy opens fire, I'm hitting the deck.

Outside the aircraft, the grunts had formed a perimeter. Overhead, the chase plane orbited, ready to swoop in and rescue us if we got dinged. Both Huey gun ships were orbiting within a few hundred yards at an altitude of eight hundred feet with their rockets and M-60s ready to hit any gook that moved.

From the distance came two grubby, unshaven grunts with muddy flak jackets draped loosely over dirty green tee shirts, running at full speed with their helmeted heads down, carrying their wounded buddy on a deeply stained olive-green stretcher. The wounded man's left pant leg was torn off and his leg was covered with a blood-soaked, mud-encrusted battle dressing.

Trying to assess the physical status of the wounded man, I leaned out the door. He was conscious. His face was pink. He was breathing. Though he had an expression of apprehension, he wasn't screaming in pain. I felt a wave of relief. This one was okay. I didn't have to do anything. We'd just transfer the guy to Charlie Med and he'd be okay. This wasn't an emergency mission, so I surmised there hadn't been any combat activity in the zone for at least an hour. I felt assured that we were going to be able to get away without any trouble.

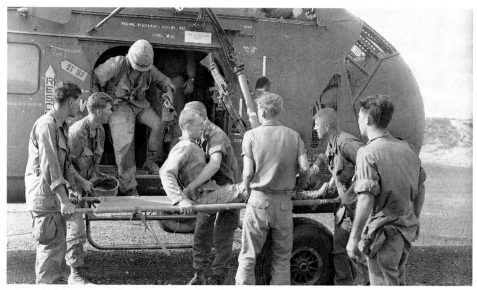

Wounded USMC soldier being loaded on UH34D for transport to Dong Ha for treatment (Source: USMC)

The guy sat up on the stretcher. We dragged him into the chopper. I helped him sit on the floor with his back to the cargo netting in the rear. That netting divided the main area of the belly from the tail, preventing us from loading the cargo too far aft of the center of gravity. Do that and the bird could flip backwards.

As the old chopper's engine revved up, everything started violently vibrating, especially my teeth. We began lifting off. It seemed to take forever to gain any altitude. Then, I felt a resurgence of fear, which I tried to dull by talking to myself again.

It's a hot day.

It's just taking a little longer to run in ground effect to finally get off.

(Silently chuckling with an image of Pam in my mind)

I wish I could get off.

(Exhaling deeply)

It's gonna be all right.

With the engine roaring at maximum R.P.M., the old bird shook worse than a paint mixer as it strained to gain altitude. Then, a huge POW! I could feel it down to the cells of my body!

What's happening?

My head was being crushed. My chest was compressed. I couldn't breathe.

What is happening?

Everything is in slow motion!

We'd been hit by enemy fire. In my mouth, I could taste magnesium, could taste gunpowder, could taste smoke. I felt fire. I looked back towards the tail compartment, and all I could see was smoke. Then I saw some daylight.

I can't hear anything!

Deafened by the concussion of the explosion, I could see that a wounded grunt was screaming. I could see his mouth open, could see his eyes bugging out, but in complete silence.

Then, the chopper started spinning.

We're out of control!

My body was reeling, as if I were floating through space, when I smashed into an ammo case. Desperately trying to steady myself, to keep from getting thrown from the aircraft, I grabbed for the grunt on the floor in front of me, to try and keep him aboard.

Then, we crashed.

My body acted autonomously, independently of my conscious mind. It displayed strength I didn't know I had, as I dragged the wounded grunt face down across the floor of the tilted chopper to the door. Stubby was already outside. We grabbed the poor son of a bitch, slinging him like a rag doll and took off in a dead run for the chase plane, which departed quickly and successfully.

Jesus, we made it out alive!

As I peered out the open door, I saw our bird – a giant ball of orange flames.

Those UH-34Ds... exploding like a lightbulb flash!

Great design, your morons!

We could have burned to death.

Goddamn!

I am fucking furious.

As we pulled out, the Hueys orbiting us laid torrents of rockets and tracers. All that shock and awe just to keep the gooks' heads down so that we could make a safe departure.

Oh yeah, baby!

Wow, we were relieved, yet all stone-faced. I noticed my flak jacket where I'd pinned a button – one of several my wife had just sent me from home. Doing a double take, I burst into tears and laughter at the same time. I passed it around. Everybody had a look, and we ended up a hysterical mob in the back of that chopper. The button? It said:

A MESSAGE FROM THE SURGEON GENERAL —
CAUTION: MILITARY SERVICE MAY BE HAZARDOUS
TO YOUR HEALTH

Deadly Fiasco Involving the M-16 Rifle

Leading up to the Vietnam war, the Army and Marines had invested in the M-16, its new combat assault rifle, designed to complete with the Soviet-built AK-47, both being lightweight and highly accurate, combining the firepower of a submachine gun with a rifle's range and accuracy.

Entering into service in the 1950s, the AK-47 was lethal, easy to use, sturdy and reliable even in the messiest of combat conditions. In the U.S., built by Colt Industries, the M-16 assault rifle was also quite

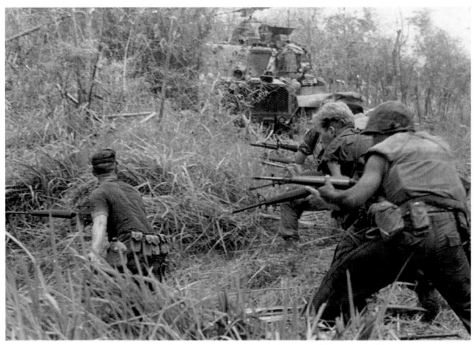

U.S. Marines aim their M-16 rifle during a battle with NVA forces (Credit: USMC)

lethal, automatically firing 5.56 mm bullets at a high velocity and blistering rate of 700 rounds per minute. Due to its small caliber, the average foot soldier can carry twice as many rounds. When the projectile hits the target, it enters as a tiny 5.56 mm hole. However, once it penetrates, the projectile tumbles, chewing up human organs and tissue.

We'll Take a Half Million

In 1966, due to its extreme lethality, the Army and Marines bought over 400,000 M-16 rifles. Within just a few months, reports began circulating about the weapon failing to feed, failing to fire and failing to extract, problems that arose from inadequate field testing, primarily due to designers with no combat experience.

For some reason – stemming from politics, economics, or ignorance – the weapon was never fully evaluated in combat conditions. If it had been, a fatal design flaw would have quickly become apparent – its shell chamber had been fashioned out of a different composition of metal from the shells themselves. Consequently, under rapid-fire conditions, as the metals swelled from the heat, differential expansion occurred. The shells became locked in the chamber, and the gun

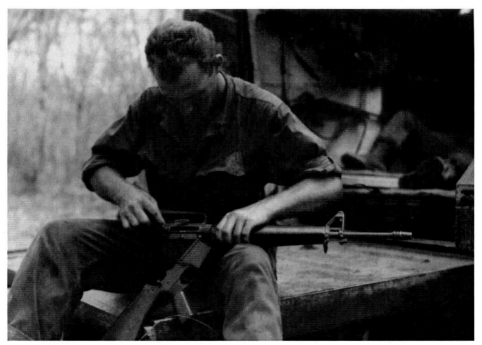
U.S. Marine cleaning his M-16 rifle (Credit: USMC)

"jammed."

The M-16 required more careful, frequent and thorough cleaning than the M-14 to function properly. The requirement was so stringent, that it was often impossible to meet in field or combat conditions. Even when the rifle was cleaned perfectly, it often failed to properly eject spent cartridges, causing a jam when the next round was chambered.

Military leaders became aware that such serious problems were arising with M-16 jams. In October of 1966, one commander admitted failures had occurred "to the extent that confidence has been downgraded."

During close-quarters battles, just like those that occurred in the Vietnam war, in a dense jungle, rainforest, marsh or beach, this flawed rifle would lead to a needless loss of U.S. Marines, with our young boys paying the ultimate price.

The Hill Fights

In the spring of 1967, at the time our infantry men were being issued the M-16s to replace their older, reliable M-14s, one of the Vietnam war's big battles was brewing. It is known as The Hill Fights, or the First Battle for Khe Sanh, the coveted remote outpost in the far northwestern corner of the country, particularly Hills 861 and 881. These outcroppings offered strategic vantage points of the area, located in terrain that was rugged and steep, covered with jungle vegetation including tree canopy, bamboo thickets and dense elephant grass.

On April 24th, five Marine grunts were scaling Hill 861 to establish an observation post. They were ambushed. Four were killed before the enemy retreated. Their squad leader called for a helicopter to evacuate the bodies. A blunt-nosed H-34, supported by gunships, spiraled down for a pick-up. As the chopper touched down, enemy machine gun fire erupted from concealed bunkers. The bird took 35 hits. As the Hueys rolled in pouring gunfire down on the hillside, the pilots made a startling discovery. They observed that the entire hilltop was honeycombed with newly constructed enemy entrenchments and huge bunkers.

Where had they all come from?

Then the attack re-ignited. In the book, *Bonnie-Sue A Marine Corps Helicopter Squadron in Vietnam*, Marion F. Sturkey, a Marine HHM-265 pilot describes how "these grunts ran into concentrated mortar attacks and machine gun fire from the entrenched North Vietnamese and a fierce battle began. Within minutes, the wounded grunts were stranded and lying helpless somewhere in the tall elephant grass between the Marine mortar positions and the NVA trenches and bunkers."

Under heavy automatic weapons fire and responding to an emergency Medevac call, a CH-46 Sea Knight, piloted by our own Jack House with co-pilot Jim Dalton, Crew Chief Lance Corporal Dan Delude and Gunner G.L. "Red" Logan was able to land with Delude dashing out and helping load the KIAs and assisting the wounded. No one was left stranded. Sturkey goes on to describe how "other casualties would not be able to make it to the helicopter without help. Dulude disconnected his long-cord, dashed out and ran 75 feet to a wounded grunt. He dragged the man back to the H-46, got him inside, and then made two more trips to retrieve wounded soldiers."

Providing cover fire, Logan recalled "just putting lots of three and four round bursts from the fifty into every place where we drew fire and I kept firing until all were in and ready to go."

Departing, Logan yelled, "It looks like an ant hill. I've never seen so many gooks."

That day, platoons from the 1st Battalion, 9th Marine Regiment (known as the Walking Dead for its high casualty rate) were sweeping caves on the hill and came under intense machine gun and mortar fire. Calling in airstrikes, unfortunately, in a friendly fire incident, an F-4 dropped two 250 lb. bombs and killed 6 Marines, mistaking them for an enemy patrol.

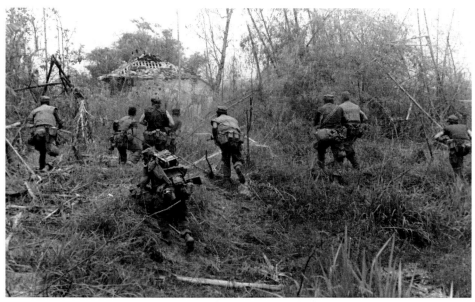

Marines rushing uphill in assault on enemy position (Credit: USMC)

The following day, in thick fog, the bloody assault on Hill 861 continued. David Petteys, one of the USMC helicopter pilots in the action recalls in his book, "A reconnaissance team was in trouble and we had to run an emergency extraction. They were taking automatic weapons and mortar fire. Five of the seven men were severely wounded. The poor kids. They sounded very frightened on the radio. They'd been hit by a mortar. They were all in shock. As our UH-1Es strafed the landing zone, I could see muzzle flashes coming at us. In the LZ, under fire, we got them aboard. Their leader thanked us profusely in tears for saving their lives."

The toll on our troops during that fight? 19 KIAs, 42 WIAs and 4 missing.

On the 27th, Petteys wrote, "We had a bird shot down. It was caught in the crossfire of .50 caliber machine guns. They're really staying and slugging it out. We've been flying loads of Medevacs. The floor of the aircraft was soaked in blood. I've seen plane load after plane load of litter/body bags fly out and C-130 loads of fresh troops being brought in."

That day, Petteys recalls an angry encounter concerning M-16 gun jams between a grunt and his commanding general on a visit to a field hospital – "One blood-soaked WIA that was brought in on a stretcher had General Hochmuth, Commanding General, 3rd Marine Division, walk up to him. The kid raised up and told the general that he wasn't going back in the field until he gave him his M-14 back and got rid of this 'piece of shit' (referring to the M-16). The kid had been face to face with an NVA when his M-16 jammed. The NVA leisurely laced him with his AK-47. He was lucky to be alive!"

His plea was not granted. The kid was ignored. Instead, the all-out assault continued.

On the 28th, artillery and air attacks were nearly continuous – 2000 rounds of 175 mm shells were fired and 518,700 lbs. of ordinance was dropped. Grunts were mounting ground assaults involving two full infantry battalions. The goal was to finally seize control of Hills 861, 881 South and finally 881 North. Gunships and Medevac helicopters waited at the Khe Sanh airstrip as the grunts swarmed up 861's steep southern slope. By nightfall, the hilltop had a new tenant.

Helicopters could land to bring water, C-rations and ammunition. Permeating the air were the rancid odors of decaying NVA bodies. Swarms of flies descended on the bloated corpses, while vultures circled overhead. Over 425 bunkers and personal fighting holes were discovered, indicating the level of resistance being encountered.

In a report about The Hill Fights by the Vietnam History Project, it describes a surprise attack that occurred on April 30th, where the Marines had been caught in a trap and "to make matters worse, their new M-16 5.56 mm riles often jammed as they tried to engage attacking NVA soldiers at close range."

A Marine platoon leader reported, "Out of the nine riflemen making the assault, six of their guns jammed almost immediately," then matter of factly recounted, "Slowed down my assault quite a bit, as the enemy was able to pick off quite a few of my men. One of our Marines had his rifle jam in the midst of a firefight and saw buddies killed while they struggled to clear blockages in the chamber of their rifle."

In that attack, there were 44 KIAs and 109 WIAs. One particular Marine company suffered 27 of those KIAs and 51 of the wounded.

Soon, the gooks became aware of our malfunctioning weapons. They'd play cat and mouse with our frantic troops. They would wait until a grunt's gun jammed and then stand up and shoot him in the lower abdomen or legs, which causes a slow and painful death. Kids came out of the field screaming, weeping and begging for better weapons.

Frantic requests for the old M-14s were nixed.

When High Command was told that the Colt M-16 rifle was jamming, their response was "Impossible!" Officers told them that the M-16 rifle was the best ever invented and the only reason it wasn't working was because they were too dumb or lazy to keep it clean.

In the early stages of this protracted battle, I was at Charlie Med in Phu Bai. On the base's flight line, I noticed two C-130s being loaded with empty body bags by the dozens. I walked over to the staff sergeant acting as load master.

"Hey, Sarge, where are those going?"

"Khe Sanh – we got caught in a shit sandwich," he hollered back.

"You mean we've lost that many guys?"

"Doc, I don't think they're enough. We're calling for more."

In the operations hootch, Charlie Pittman was reviewing operations of the day. I came in to inquire: "Hey Charlie, what's happening up there?"

"They're in a world of hurt. Far as we know here, 1/9 was running routine patrols at the DMZ when one bunch of guys encountered the enemy in a valley between hills 881 and 861 just northwest of Khe Sanh. At first, we thought they were a band of Cong locals. Our guys called for reinforcements and got sent a platoon, and they were outnumbered. Now a couple of companies are working the area and they're calling for more. We figure the gooks have a whole division of North Vietnamese Army. We've got our hands full. We're pulling 'em out of the field by the dozens. Heard something about their guns jamming."

"Who's flying the Medevacs up there?" I asked. "Sperb and Newcomb. Doc Bohiman's still at Dong Ha, but we're probably gonna need him soon. I gotta run now. You stay back here just in case you're needed later. Don't come now," he called over his shoulder as he and his crew hurried out to their chopper. I sat around the ready room bullshitting with the guys and playing acey-ducey, when around lunch time a call came in. One of the majors that I knew only as a nodding acquaintance came up to me. "Doc, I hate to ask this, but can you go to Khe Sanh? They just lost their medical officer."

His name was Donald Linker, the 1/9's GMO, General Medical Officer. He'd been sent to Khe Sanh's medical bunker to deliver emergency care.

"What happened?"

"He cracked from exhaustion. He'd been up thirty-six hours straight in the bunker and they brought in KIAs and WIAs by the dozens. He didn't stop. He never left the bunker. He even pissed himself. Finally, he just collapsed. They just Medevac'd him out. There's no doctor up there. Will you go?" he asked.

Called into the Mayhem

"Sure." I replied.

I'm exhausted running Medevacs.

At least, I'd be stationary.

At a full run, I grabbed my gear and jumped aboard a C-130 re-supply mission to Khe Sanh, which was about twenty minutes away. In its storage area, the bird had stacks upon stacks of ammunition and multiple bundles of body bags.

Wow.

Stacks of ammunition boxes.

Bundles of body bags.

We empty one.

And fill the other.

Landing in Khe Sanh, an active war zone, this big cargo bird had to make a steep dive for the runway, hit the tarmac with a controlled crash and immediately throw the props in full reverse and slam on the

176

brakes. It's a thrill ride with those last few yards of landing, always a white-knuckles skid in a cloud of red dust.

As our aircraft came to a halt, the large aft ramp dropped. Looking outside from the cargo hold, I could see nothing. Visibility was zero in the billowing red dust. I gathered my equipment and made my way out. As the choking cloud dissipated, I could see grunts in helmets and flak jackets scurrying around, dumping what appeared to be bulky sandbags along the sides of the runway. I was wrong. They were dead Marines. Most were in body bags, but others with just ponchos over them, and a few with no covering at all – all stacked motionless like cordwood.

Our Combat Hospital Bunker

Covered with the red dust of Vietnam, carrying the stench of death, gunpowder and jet fumes, I ran towards the bunker that served as Khe Sanh's medical facility. It was a large structure, about twenty by forty feet, dug into the ground so that its walls were mud for about six feet up, with sand bags above that for another three feet, with a tin roof overhead.

I fit right in.

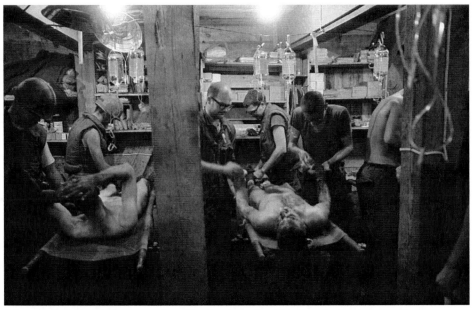

Wounded soldiers being treated at Khe Sanh medical bunker during intense close contact fighting (Credit: USMC)

This crude field hospital was divided into two rooms, one for triage and the other for surgery. Strewn about in front of the bunker's entrance lay at least forty litters containing the wounded and dead. Corpsmen ran from litter to litter, calling out wound assessments. I'd just joined the grisly mayhem that drove the last doctor out of his mind.

As I approached, one of the corpsmen sprinted towards me and grabbed my bags. "Doc, we're triaging the wounded in front here. The good ones can sit it out until we can get 'em back to Danang in the C-130s. They're only bringing a couple of birds an hour and the choppers are busy in the field. We need you to look at the bad ones – decide who's salvageable, who's not. For the guys dying, we'll need to shoot them up with morphine to make'm comfortable. We're taking the KIAs to the airfield. Hold your breath when you go in the bunker, it's really putrid in there."

He was right. When I entered the bunker, a foul stench rose up before my nostrils – the odor of dried blood, gunpowder, piss, shit, sweat, and death. The floor was slimy with entrails, intestines, shit, and blood strewn from one end to the other. At least fifteen litters, each with a severely wounded marine, sat in that slime. The corpsman working in the bunker saw me looking at the guts on the floor and explained, "The doctor had to cut a few feet of gut out to keep a grunt from bleeding out. The guy will make it. In Danang, they'll put a colostomy in him." He turned to start an IV and mumbled, "Actually, we've had to do it on a couple of guys. We just can't get to cleaning up. Fuckin' M-16! Fuckin M-16!" Then he turned to me and asked, "Doc, will you check those five guys over there?"

Gooks Opened Up on Us – Couldn't Do Nothing

One of this group of five was a burly young redhead with blue-green eyes, barely old enough to grow any beard, which sprouted as a short stubble from his chin. Grubby and dirty, he looked at me with his wide eyes filled with tears and said, "Doc, it was terrible. We were on this ridge. There were ten of us. All of a sudden, these gooks start comin' up the side of the ridge. I can't tell you, but there couldn't have been more than five or six of them. They all had AK-47s. We had these

178

fuckin' M-16s."

"Anyway, we opened up on 'em and surprised 'em. I nailed one right in the head. But then my gun jammed. My fuckin' gun jammed. And then my buddy's gun jammed. And then, damn near all of us had our guns jammin' on us. Fuckin' things! They just wouldn't work. We hit the ground. The fuckin' gooks looked over and saw us and they started laughing. They were just walking, standing straight up, walking straight at us, laughing their asses off, pointing their guns at us."

"We couldn't do nothin', Doc, we couldn't do nothin'. The fuckin' guns wouldn't work. I threw my fuckin' gun at one of 'em, hopin' I could kill the son of a bitch. Didn't hit him. Couldn't do nothin'. Then the gooks opened up on us. They opened up on us. We had no fuckin' rifles. We had nothin'. Killed a lot of us. I'm gonna be okay, ain't I, Doc? Ain't I gonna be okay? I made it, didn't I?"

Peering into his eyes , I reassured him, "Yeah, kid, it's all right. You're gonna be okay."

When I opened up the battle dressing on his gut, I saw the three massive exit wounds the AK-47 shells had made at short range – one right under the navel, another just to the right of that, about two inches higher, and the third in his right flank. I could see the blood and innards pulsing underneath the macerated skin. I didn't bother to turn the kid over. I knew by the trajectory of the exit wounds that the entry wounds were high. He had been shot while he lay helpless on his belly. His left leg was totally limp and his left foot turned inward at ninety degrees to his right foot. I knew that meant one bullet had shattered his spine, because I couldn't see any wounds around his legs. I was sure he had flaccid paralysis of that left leg.

I didn't bother to go any further: I knew the kid couldn't survive. The only way we could have even thought about salvaging him was to have at least four units of blood to pump into him immediately, and then we'd have to perform four or five hours of sophisticated bowel surgery to save any of his gut. That level of medical treatment was at least two hours away, and looking at him, he wasn't going to last more than twenty minutes.

For a brief moment, in all of the chaos, my mind flashed back to the real world, where I'd been trained in shock trauma medicine – the pristine emergency rooms with consultants to spare. There, I never felt alone. I could always call someone who knew exactly what to do. The worst we'd see would be a couple of auto accident victims. It was actually exciting. It was fun. When I needed blood replacement, all I did was order it. Everything got done. When the patient needed surgery, we always had an abundance of surgical residents hungry for the experience of cutting on someone. Anesthesiologists stood ready to intubate and administer anesthetics. We had laboratories to perform pre-operative blood tests. We had fully-equipped operating rooms. The lights stayed on. No fading in and out with the surges of a cranky field generator. The floors weren't dirt, the ceilings weren't rusty tin.

This place where I found myself looked and smelled worse than a shuttered slaughterhouse. There was nothing I could do to help a dying soldier in this hole. I looked at him and nodded, "Yeah, kid, you're gonna be all right." I gave him thirty milligrams of morphine in one intramuscular injection and had the corpsman carry his stretcher over to a corner of the room so he could die in peace.

As helicopters continued delivering the wounded and dead from the field, I'd triage them, ordering that the more severely wounded be carried into the medical bunker for some definitive initial treatment that might allow them to survive the flight by C-130 back to Danang and into the much more sophisticated hospital complex there.

Too often, I was pronouncing guys dead. Their lifeless bodies were hauled off to join their buddies laying outside. I hoped that I wouldn't make a mistake and pronounce a salvageable, a living guy, as deceased.

I will never know for sure. That still haunts me.

While placing a tourniquet and battle dressing on a leg, I asked the corpsman helping me, "What's this about the M-16?"

"It's the new rifle they issued the grunts a few weeks ago. Took away their M-14s. Lucky I didn't give up my M-14." He re-directed the conversation. "Doc, Lou needs your help with that guy over there," pointing to a lanky corpsman, working on a grunt with large battle dressings on his head and abdomen.

Lou looked up with bloodshot eyes sunk into a hollow face that displayed a stubble of beard, cracked lips and dried saliva which made whitish crusts at the corners of his mouth. He was another beleaguered corpsman, who'd been up for days, appearing just like the rest of these guys – walking corpses.

"Doc, what should I do with him?" he asked, pointing to the wounded grunt on the litter in front of him.

This Marine looked cleaner than most.

Must be a replacement.

Newbie. Poor sucker.

Got hit bad.

Over his face, this guy had large battle dressing covering his left eye and side of his head. His right eye was open, the pupil dilated. I reached over to a wooden table against the wall of the bunker and picked up an opthalmoscope. Shining it into the eye caused no pupiliary response. I touched his eye, and the lid closed by reflex. I thought to myself – the pupil is fixed and dilated and I get a corneal reflex. What's going on? Next I checked his breathing. Someone had placed a plastic airway in his mouth and trachea, and he breathed regularly, unlabored. It looked to me like he was suffering from traumatic brain edema.

Then I looked under the dressing on his head. The entire left frontal bone had been shattered by the bullet's exit wound. He had been shot in the back of the head. No eye remained – the eye socket gaped, shattered and eviscerated. The left frontal lobe of his brain was laid open and shattered, the left hemisphere behind it covered with a massive clot of blood. I shuddered and replaced the battle dressing over the wound.

"Forget it. This guy's had it. Why don't you carry him in front of the bunker and let him go in peace?" I suggested, as Lou began to well up with tears. The young corpsman himself worried me.

"What about you?" I asked him. "Have you eaten or slept lately?"

"Don't worry, Doc. I got three or four hours of shut-eye last night. I'll be all right," he answered between low choking sobs.

"Doc! Doc! Over here!" came the cry from a corpsman in the far corner as he began pounding on the chest of a prostrate grunt.

I turned and ran to the grunt, who appeared to have a massive wound in his right arm. A flimsy battle dressing fell off revealing that the flesh on the lateral half of his arm had been blown away. The muscles around the bone, the humerus, lay exposed. The arm had been broken completely in two, with the shattered stumps fully exposed and bleeding.

"He's lost a lot of blood, but we can save him," the corpsman concluded.

"Let's get a couple of pints of albumin running into him. Get one in the left arm, the other in his foot. Open him up wide," I hollered.

Three of the corpsmen dropped what they were doing and ran over to assist. While they started IVs and CPR, I tended to the arm wound, first placing a tourniquet on the upper aspect of the arm. As I worked on it, the lower part of the arm fell off the litter and yanked the dressings away from my hands. I realized that the arm was hanging by only a few muscles and strands of flesh. The fingers had already turned so blue the circulation in the lower aspect of that limb had to be nonexistent. The arm was no good. I grabbed a scalpel and severed the last few pieces of flesh that held it to the upper stump, caught hold of the severed arm and placed it between the man's legs. Then I was able to put a neat, tight pressure dressing on the stump to stop further oozing. The IVs were running full bore, the heart had started beating, the breathing was regular, and the man had begun to regain consciousness.

"I think he's going to make it," I told the corpsman.

"All right!" he shouted, smiling and thrusting his fist into the air as all of the other corpsman began to cheer.

"You guys are doing a great job," I told the team. "We have to watch this guy closely, but I think he'll survive. Be sure to ship the arm down with him, just in case we've got a super surgeon at NSA or on the Repose who wants to try to sew it back on."

One of the corpsmen turned to start working on another wounded grunt and mumbled, "Fuckin' M-16."

I went over to evaluate him. The boy had both feet filled with shrapnel. Apparently, he had caught an antipersonnel round to the lower portion of his body. I needed to inspect him for shrapnel. As I started cutting his pants off, the corpsman volunteered, "Let me do that, Doc."

"Okay, I'll get an IV going." The grunt was awake and breathing but looked too scared to talk. In fact, he looked terrified and catatonic.

"It's a million-dollar wound, guy. You're okay," I reassured him.

As I worked on the IV, I struck up a conversation with the corpsman while inspecting the lower trunk and legs. "What's going on with the M-16?" I inquired.

"It's jammin', Doc. It don't work. It ain't worth shit in combat," he answered. "They issued it to the grunts a few weeks ago. Took away their M-14s."

"Why'd they do that?"

"The 16's a new rifle. It's from Colt. You know – they make the 45. Anyway, it's supposed to be a better weapon. The only problem is it's jammin'. Just when the grunt needs his rifle most, it jams. The gooks carry them Russian AK-47s. They're as good as the old 14. You could drop 'em in the water and still fire 'em. With the fuckin' 16, our guys are outclassed," he grumbled.

"The kids keep crying," he told me as he finished up on the grunt's leg. "They want their 14s back. The general says no. They keep sending up replacements with them fuckin' 16s, and they keep comin' back in body bags. The general says the 16's good. They got to use it."

"Why do you think they won't give the 14s back?" I asked.

"I don't know. Maybe the general owns a lot of stock in Colt Industries," the corpsman suggested.

"From what I've heard about this fucking war so far, I wouldn't put it past him," I muttered to him as I went back to check on the big redhead. He was dead. "Move him up to the runway. Be sure to bring back the litter," I shouted to a corpsman who seemed to be free at the moment.

Then I moved on to care for another trooper with a big gaping wound in his right calf. The leg probably would have to be amputated, but I elected to put a pressure dressing on it, splint it, and start an IV.

"Hey, Doc. I know how we can win this war," he chuckled in his pain. "I got a secret weapon."

"Oh yeah? What is it?" I smiled as I started an IV in his arm.

"It's the M-16. A gook stole a 16 from one of our KIAs and took it into his spider hole. When he popped up to ambush us, he got only five or six rounds off before it jammed. We laced his ass. I think we should issue all the gooks these M-16s and take our 14s back. Then we'd have this war over in a hurry."

All day and night, the wounded and dead streamed in. The word was that three out of four had been killed because their rifles had jammed. Finally, morning came and with it a C-130 carrying my blessed replacement. I welcomed the new medical officer whom I never met with a big hug.

"Man, am I glad to see you!"

"Really? I heard about what's been happening up here. How's it going now?" he asked.

"Seems to be slowing down. Are there still KIAs lining the runway?" I asked. I hadn't been out of the bunker in at least eight hours.

"Pretty much, pretty much," he answered with a weak voice. "What's going on here?"

"Butcher shop stuff, man, just butcher shop stuff. All you can do is stop the bleeding, maintain an open airway, and start IVs. We're pretty well supplied with everything but litters and body bags. I guess those will come later when this thing calms down. Okay if I split now? I've had it."

"Yeah, go ahead. The C-130 out there's going back to Marble. They're offloading the WIAs directly to NSA. Grab it."

When that flight, loaded with the wounded, landed at Marble Mountain, I went to the squadron's hootch and collapsed in a spare cot, fully clothed, and slept all the rest of the day and through the night.

Heading Straight for the Commanding Officer

When I awoke the next morning, I only had one thing on my mind. I didn't want to eat or clean-up. All I wanted was to get to a MAG commander and report on the M-16 issues and how our boys were getting cut down. The closest headquarters was G-3, which was stenciled in gold letters over the doors I barged through, startling two captains in the midst of their morning Cup of Joe. That phrase was actually coined by Navy sailors, shortened from a Cup of Joseph Daniels, the Navy Secretary under President Woodrow Wilson. It was meant as a disparaging remark about coffee, served with greater frequency due to the Secretary's campaign to improve military morals, which included a reduction in prostitution and a ban on alcohol.

So, the guys were drinking their coffee, when I confronted them. "I'm Levin. Just got back from Khe Sanh. I'm reporting about the M-16 rifle jams. It's wiping out our grunts."

The two men looked at me – unshaven, my flight suit encrusted with dried blood – and immediately responded. "We'll take you to the G-2, Colonel Melton," said one. "He's the base intelligence officer."

He grabbed me by the arm and led me out of the hootch to the one next door. Inside, we hurried past the stunned captain sitting at the desk in the front and into the back room. There in his office, was Colonel Melton, a short man with sandy blond hair, puffing on a cigar.

"What's wrong, Captain Hart?" he asked my escort.

'The Doc here's from Khe Sanh. He wants to tell you something."

"Okay, Doc, have a seat." He pointed to a chair in front of his desk. As I sat down I noticed a chalk board behind the colonel: "Khe Sanh – 340 KIA, 1263 WIA."

With an obvious look of agitation, I excitedly described how the "1/9 got wiped out up there. We lost a lot of guys. Their rifles are jamming. They're being shot point-blank because their guns didn't work. We've got to do something. They're screaming for their M-14s."

"Doctor," the colonel retorted with a blazing stare, "You're distraught, you've been working too hard. Take some time off."

"Colonel, I saw it with my own eyes." Pointing to the board, I proclaimed, "These numbers can't be right. I processed at least three times that many."

The colonel looked at me with fire in his eyes and answered, "There were three hundred forty men killed in that operation, soldier, and that's the number you'll live with, or else."

I squirmed uneasily in my chair and looked at the two captains standing in the room.

"And besides that, Doctor", he declared, "The M-16 rifle works just fine. Have you got that?"

The Colonel rose from behind his desk, puffing his cigar, looking down at me like a Dutch uncle. He added, "Doc, let me give it to you straight. I'm a Naval Academy graduate. I'm a colonel in the Marine Corps. I'm up for general, and I don't want to lose that promotion. Have you got it?"

The younger captain came to my chair, put his hand on my shoulder and said,

"Let it go, Doc. Just let it go."

"Okay, I will," I sternly replied.

I did. I let it go.

A couple of weeks later when I was at Phu Bai, Bill Sperb came running up to me. "Hey Doc, did you hear that Congress is conducting a big investigation about the M-16 fiasco? They're testing the M-16 at the Aberdeen Proving Ground in Maryland. The fuckin' gun's gonna jam on 'em, and we're gonna get our 14s back. Just wait and see."

"Lots of luck, Bill! I'll believe it when I see it."

Blame the Grunts

One day as I walked into the operations bunker Bill grabbed my arm.

"Did you hear about General Green?" he asked. "He testified before Congress that the reason why the 16 jams is because we're too fuckin' dumb to keep it clean. Can you beat that shit? We're too fuckin' dumb to keep it clean," he taunted angrily.

Then he began to play-act, casting himself as General Green. "General, sir, we all know you're a good soldier and you can keep your weapons clean, but we bad soldiers get dirty in combat, sir."

"Yeah!" chimed in Fred Newcomb, going along with the act. "How come you can't keep your fatigues pressed or your boots shined in combat? Why, I remember when I was in combat. I kept my brass polished, my fatigues cleaned and pressed, and my shoes shined. You assholes can't even keep your guns clean."

"When was you in combat sir?" Sperb archly inquired.

"Uh, let me see, son. I guess it was in one of those John Wayne movies or something,"

Newcomb pontificated as the entire roomful of grunts broke up in laughter. When things quieted down, I puzzled, "You'd think that the field trials would have shown them that the guns jammed."

"Doc, the field trials were at 881," Newcomb soberly responded. "Remember, it's the only war we have. Make it last."

Unbeknownst to us, back Stateside, there was a massive effort underway to regrind and re-plate the rifle chambers with a new metal. After that, new M-16s coming online had re-bored and chrome-plated chambers that reduced the differential expansion between the chamber and the projectile. Apparently, there had been more than just dirt that had jammed the guns.

I was furious that the American public swallowed their bullshit explanation, blaming our brave boys. Following this fiasco, our morale plummeted. While we just survived a hellish nightmare, where many of our buddies were helplessly killed, we were also confronted with objective evidence that we were being used as pawns. A crudely lettered sign showed up outside the grunts' compound. It proclaimed:

United States Marines:
The Unwilling
Led by the Incompetent
To Do the Impossible
For the Ungrateful.

Our high command had failed us. Now we felt all alone. And we were angry.

In his book, David Petteys wrote in May of 1967, "The war grinds on. This 'measured response' baloney is ridiculous. We are fighting battle after battle over the same terrain and not proving or settling a thing. And, of course, we're paying with plane loads of dead 19-year-olds. The NVA is moving back into Hill 881, north of Khe Sanh, so all the ground we won, at the expense of 300 KIA and 900 WIA, is going back to Charlie. No kidding! The reconnaissance teams see them building bunkers. Useless!"

Nobody gave a damn. We were painfully aware of that.

For us, it was all about each other.

Chapter Ten
My Complete Psychotic Break-Down

*"I saw battle corpses, myriads of them, And the white skeletons of young men,
I saw them; But I saw they were not as was thought, They themselves were
fully at rest; they suffered not; The living remain'd and suffer'd."*
Walt Whitman

Being truly heroic, risking death or injury for others with no regard for personal safety, amazes us when someone displays such actions. One might ponder, "How did they do that?" Another could respond, "I'm not that brave." Or, "That person must have been out of their mind."

Well, he or she just may have been.

I was.

On the night of September 12, 1967, during Operation Wheeler/Wallowa, Nui Loc Son, a company of U.S. Marines, 2nd Battalion, 4th Regiment, 3rd Marine Division, nicknamed the "Magnificent Bastards," were pinned down by enemy fire. Some had been killed. Many others were badly wounded. Ammunition was running critically short. A frantic call came into the Dong Ha base for an emergency Medevac and re-supply.

I was there. I didn't have to, but I volunteered for the special mission.

WHOP-WHOP-WHOP

As our bird was approaching the LZ, loaded with wood pallets of rifle ammo, grenades, mortar shells and medical supplies, we came under intense enemy fire. Rockets and mortars were flying around us, missing their target, but exploding upon impact. We were forced to back out, aborting our landing. We tried again. We were forced back out again. On the third occasion, we didn't land, but touched the ground and slowly taxied. While our crew chief and gunner fired their machine guns, the back door opened, and I began pushing these pallets out and onto the ground.

I was scared shitless.

Somehow, I also wound up outside the aircraft. I either jumped or fell. Once on the ground, I noticed the scores of dead and wounded. Our helo was departing. I could've escaped. I chose not to. Crazy? Probably. Instead of jumping back on board, I scurried for a foxhole with gunfire raging around me. One of the Marines there with me tried to climb out to help his badly wounded buddy, who was nearby and screaming in pain. I grabbed his flak jacket and forcibly pulled him down. My attention turned to treating the wounded, soon finding out their corpsman had been killed. So, I was the lone medical person there.

Then, I heard a loud machine gun burst with bullets flying overhead.

RATTA-TAT-TAT

That damn grunt, who tried to get up, did so while I wasn't paying attention. That volley had blown him to pieces with body parts laying everywhere. Poor bastard should've heeded my warning and kept his head down. But, as a U.S. Marine, true to Semper Fi, he refused to abandon his buddy, even if it cost him his life.

Turning back to the wounded, some were clearly near death, so I administered morphine syrettes to end their suffering. I always hung several of these on my flak jacket, because I frequently needed them. Nobody ever stole one from me.

I treated others who had a chance at survival. I was able to intubate a Marine with a horrible facial wound. I hung IV bags. I applied pressure dressings. All night, we were under relentless attack, but kept our survivors alive. Fortunately, we had Huey gunships flying over us, reining hell upon the enemy, thwarting their continuous advances.

I got out safely the next day.

Later, I was informed by the Awards Officer that I would be receiving a Silver Star for heroism, citing me with a "...display of exceptional courage above and beyond the call of duty in keeping with the highest traditions of the Marine Corps and of the United States Naval Service and undoubtedly saving the lives of many Marines. For the President, V. H. Krulak, U.S. Marine Corps Commanding General, Fleet Marine Force, Pacific."

Hey General! Remember me? You wanted me court-martialed for criticizing how we were throwing our kids away with stupid battle tactics and defective weapons that in the heat of battle won't fire.

On that occasion, I wasn't honored by my commendation, but intensely angry. Having made it out of there alive, I felt terribly guilty. It flogged my mind.

Yet, when a Medevac call came. I suspended everything else. I acted on instinct. I was a healer, for sure, but also a fighter. In Vietnam, I had been honed into a seasoned trauma doctor and highly skilled killer.

On September 19, 1967, I was aboard a CH-53 with the HMM 463 on a Medevac mission. Exiting the landing zone, we came under fire. The crew chief firing the .50 cal next to me took a round in his left wrist. He couldn't continue firing. I stopped what I was doing and looked outside. There were dozens of young gooks, many of whom looked no older than 14 years of age, shooting at us. I saw the muzzle flashes. I heard the rapid pows. This was life and death, I knew that. It was us or them. I grabbed the handles of the machine gun, took aim and pulled the trigger, mowing them down. My crew yelled out, "You got'm!" I was in shock.

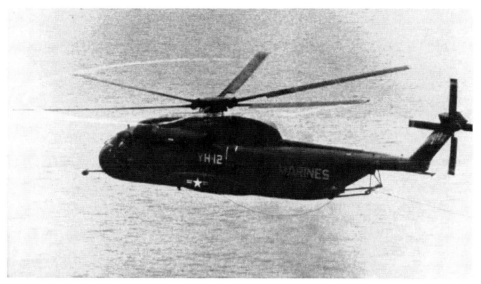

Marine CH-53 helicopter on airborne mission (Credit: USMC)

It was them or you!

Then, in a sudden mentally destructive realization…

I am a pediatrician, killing children.

As a person, I'd been bifurcated – a healer and a killer. I was able to throw a switch between both sides. I could deliver emergency medical care under extreme conditions focusing on saving lives, while also being able to mercilessly eradicate our enemies, whoever they were, without reserve or hesitation when called upon to do so. Control your terror. Crush any natural resistance to killing. Do your job. Get out alive. Bring your team back with you. Bury any moral objections that might arise.

Or, at least, try to manage the aftermath of CQB (Close Quarters Battle) and what actions you took in performing your duties. Mentally, it made me quite ill. My overall attitude toward life changed completely. Those last vestiges of the bright young man, who had done so well in medical school, in research and as a postdoctoral fellow with ambitions of becoming an astronaut – those dreams had shriveled and died, or at least reduced to life support.

I had become a cold, bitter and angry man.

Physically, I had wasted away.

Before Vietnam, I had been a fitness buff, always enjoying being strong and agile. At five foot ten, I entered the military weighing a hundred eighty-five pounds. Back then, I had the nickname, "Big Al" with a bull neck and bulging arms. I prided myself in being able to do twenty-five push-ups with one hand then shift to the other for twenty-five more. I could readily get down and do several hundred sit ups with no trouble. In pre-flight training on the obstacle course, I kept up with the best of them and set a record for the mile swim wearing a flight suit.

I was strong and virile.

Within a few months in Vietnam, I'd lost it all. My skin had become sallow and dry, my eyes sunken and hollow. My clothes draped on me, but since I wore flight suits and fatigues, this loss of body mass only became noticeable to me while on leave. I noticed my peacetime uniforms seemed to be getting bigger on me. Even my hat grew too large. I was shriveling. My weight had plummeted. All I wanted was sleep – any time I could, I would collapse. I had become morose and depressed, completely devoid of sexual interest or drive.

Worst of all, I envied the dead.

Pinned with decorations, the wounded returned home with physical disabilities, deformities and mental illnesses as their trophies of war. I felt at the time that the dead were lucky. They had won, buried with honor and fondly remembered. Benefits flowed to families, who processed their loss through the stages of grief and moved forward.

For most, there was closure.

During my tour of duty, doing my job, seeing all of our dead soldiers, I often marveled at how calm they looked. No more fear, no more suffering, no need to go home to face the denigration and hostility of an ungrateful nation. Those that perished in the war didn't have to hack it anymore, and I envied them.

I was alive but broken. My psyche was busted into pieces. I was not me.

In Vietnam, I suffered greatly from the continuous psychic shocks to my brain: my first kill of a teenaged enemy soldier, the needless suffering of our troops due to a defective rifle and the loss of a dear comrade and friend who had burned to death. All of those memories voraciously tormented me. They played over and over in my mind, inflicting deep mental lacerations and causing searing pain. It built up within me, casualty after casualty.

Emotionally, I'd become encrusted like thick scar tissue. No guilt. No remorse. Just kill or be killed. Every time one of my fellow doctors, pilots, corpsmen and friends died, I'd volunteer to go out on a mission, hoping to kill a few gooks. I became so notorious that my squadron mates spoke with pride about their bloodthirsty quack who could blow the enemy away like any salty Marine grunt with a great aim and amazing reflexes.

Surviving combat is nothing to boast about – no noble action, no glorious feat. It's the contrary. It's the ability to desensitize oneself from most of the values anyone embraces in order to contribute to a civilized society. Experiencing combat quickly conditions you to the terror-filled awareness that they are out to get you.

Your enemy wants you dead.

Period.

We were the intruders, the bad guys. This was not a political or ideological debate to them. This was a game for keeps.

You go crazy trying cope with what is being demanded of you. I did.

I'll Get Those Damn Bastards

Before I arrived in Vietnam, I was never hostile, violent or exhibited a lack of respect or self-control. Obviously, that changed. While in-country, word got around that a group of politicians were on tour, including several Senators and Congressmen. They had a familiar modus operandi, always basing themselves at large, secure military faculties like Saigon and Danang, where they availed themselves of fine wines, caviar and prostitutes.

Commanders would be forewarned and ordered to round up several hundred boys from each politician's constituency, lining them up on the landing strip for an arrival ceremony. Their fancy airplane, a twin-engine Caribou, would fly into the base. They'd disembark with a photographer strategically placed in front them. Then, the boys would stream past for their pictures to be taken as the politicians took to their glad-handing.

They'd spend a few minutes doing that, and then having grabbed their press shots, would scurry off back to their posh accommodations. Usually, only troopers who were new arrivals attended these ceremonies. The seasoned grunts hated politicians. They remained upset about the M-16 fiasco and angry that it was easier to get supplies from the black market than from their own legitimate sources. Combat-hardened troopers viewed the United States government as the worst threat to them.

I couldn't wait for the sleazeballs to come to Phu Bai – that would finally present me with the opportunity to take down somebody I really didn't like. Up until then, everybody I'd killed was somebody I really had no grudge against. Now, I could finally shoot a nice fat, sloppy, cowardly American politician right in the jelly-belly and watch him vomit his crepes and champagne.

To me, that would have been awesome! Everybody at the base knew I was psychotic. Nobody reacted, though. They kept details of the visit under wraps to help reduce any threats from their lunatic flight surgeon.

As I walked around the base, everybody was looking at me funny. Something was wrong, but I didn't know quite what it was. I kept on asking the fellows, "What's going on? What are you guys keeping from me?" They all laughed or chuckled and walked away. Finally, one of the corpsman on duty at the dispensary broke down.

"They're here," he replied forthrightly and with some disgust.

"You mean those pigs from Washington?"

"Yeah, they're here."

My face flushed red. My mind snapped. I bolted from the dispensary and ran towards the operations hootch. I stole the operations officer's Jeep. I had no time to gather up weapons. All I had with me was my little .38 special. I roared down the dirt roads through our compound, around the landing strip, and through the access road just as our guests were taking off. I'd missed them, but I didn't care. I sped after them anyway, at this point, trailing about a hundred and fifty yards behind the Caribou as it lifted off. I still fired my .38, madly obsessing on that bird coming down.

It wasn't going to happen. I was much too far away. I'm now thankful it didn't. Life in the brig was not in my thoughts in those insane moments, observed by all the guys at the landing strip who were laughing their asses off at their fanatical quack who'd now run his Jeep into the drainage ditch.

I was a certifiable lunatic.

Chapter Eleven
Joining the CIA's Covert War

"A war in which each soldier fought for his own life and the lives of the men beside him, not caring how he killed or how many or in what manner and feeling only contempt for those who sought to impose on his savage struggle the mincing distinctions of civilized warfare, the code of battlefield ethics that attempted to humanize an essentially inhuman war."

Philip Caputo
A Rumor of War
Holt Rinehart and Winston
1978

In escalating the Vietnam War, by 1967, we were bringing the power of shock and awe.

From the air, we bombed enemy forces and infrastructure into oblivion. We'd engaged in fierce fighting with the NVA and Viet Cong on the ground. To weaken them, we destroyed their infrastructure – villages, crops and livestock – implementing the widespread spraying of defoliants that was progressively laying waste to the countryside. Our strategy was to deflate our enemy's capability by depriving them of potential resources and recruits.

When asked about civilian casualties caused by our bombing and shelling, a senior general commented, "Yes, it is a problem, but it does deprive the enemy of the population, doesn't it?"

Reports concerning civilian casualties in the Vietnam war estimated that as a result of "friendly" military action, at least 150,000 were killed and 350,000 were wounded or maimed.

Refugee Crisis

Due to the war, approximately 5 million South Vietnamese civilians had become refugees, nearly a third of their population. In the villages and camps, people were dying of malnutrition and babies were being born deformed. In the cities, where there was no sanitation and rarely any running water, people were dying of cholera, typhoid, smallpox, leprosy and bubonic plague. The children succumbed to such diseases as scabies and skin sores.

In the midst of the humanitarian crises, U.S. Navy and Marine medical personnel delivered services to impacted civilian populations, in an effort to supposedly win "hearts and minds." For us, it was a means to re-connect ourselves to a sense of family, and our presence being beneficial and not hostile.

We poured tons of support into the country. In addition to our military presence and its impact on local economies, massive amounts of direct domestic aid flowed in – food, drugs, tools, construction materials, household supplies, seeds, land mines and enough barbed wire to circle the country an estimated 17 times. We knew at the time that not all of the money would be going to where it was supposed to. We figured that about 25% of the funds would be siphoned off by corrupt South Vietnamese officials and another 25% would be wasted.

Our Secret War on Civilians

America spent heavily aiding civilians. We also targeted some of them as part of CIA covert counter-insurgency campaigns, including clandestine military operations, directed specifically at civilians who were Communist members or supporters. It became known as Operation Phoenix. Run by the South Vietnamese, the CIA provided technical and logistical capabilities including Air America, its own air force and the use of trained personnel from the Army Special Forces.

According to the MACV Directive 381-41, the intent of the program was to attack the VC "with a rifle shot rather than a shotgun approach." Its goal was to eliminate the Viet Cong Infrastructure (VCI), by targeting civilian leaders and their families.

Overall, there were an estimated 81,000 arrests and interrogations, 33,000 were sent to prison, 26,000 killed and 22,000 changed allegiances. The program was reported as "highly effective." However, it was also criticized for its tactics involving interrogation, torture and assassinations.

On June 3, 1967, one of my best pilot buddies, Captain Stephen P.

Hanson had volunteered, along with his crew, to participate in a CIA Air America mission to extract a Special Forces team in Laos which was attached to a joint service high command unconventional warfare task force. These teams were performing deep penetration missions of strategic reconnaissance and interdiction.

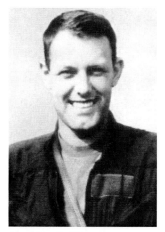

Stephen P. Hanson
Major (Posthumous)
Marine Aircraft Wing 36
USMC

Shortly into their mission, a call came that Steve's copter had taken enemy fire and needed emergency medical assistance. At that time, Dave McAllister and I were flying a routine Medevac into the Khe Sanh area. But since the call was for one of our own guys, we had to go.

So, we diverted from our intended landing zone.

Nervously, I prepared myself. We were in a CH-46A chopper, a relatively fast bird, so the trip took less than fifteen minutes. Of course, the border between Vietnam and Laos was unmarked, and the terrain was the same, so I was disoriented as to exactly where we were heading. Then we began to circle, looking for the downed choppers. We saw a puff of white smoke rising from a large clearing in the jungle, and a burning chopper. It was Steve's 46, down but intact.

What had happened? Why couldn't he make it out of there? Just about then, our chopper jolted to the right and began a steep descent into the zone. Charlie the crew chief punched my shoulder. "You and me are going in to look this over. We got to move fast. It's motherfuckin' hot down there," he shouted. I knew he wasn't referring to the ambient temperature, so I double-checked my .38 and tapped at my survival knife – double insurance.

Our bird hit the ground, we jumped out of the door and ran for Steve's chopper thirty yards away. When we got there, we saw Steve lying slumped over the forward control panel and the copilot sitting with his head cocked back against the window. The shattered windscreen and large-caliber holes forming a line across the cockpit's rear bulkhead made it obvious that the gooks had opened up on them, point blank, while they were on the ground. Body parts were strewn everywhere. The chopper was riddled with large caliber holes. No way any of these guys still could have been alive.

"Nobody here," hollered Charlie. "What you got up there?"

'These guys are dead! No way we can help. Let's get the hell out of here!" I shouted back.

We both sprinted back to our chopper at full speed and by some miracle drew no fire as we lifted off. Returning safely, I felt a violent rage. Why did these guys have to die? Back at base, people chuckled at my naivete.

Frank Miller shouted, "Wake up, Doc! This shit is about the CIA's own private war. They've got to pay for it. They need that black money. Heroin brings in big bucks. Look at the British and their opium wars. How the fuck do you think Hong Kong became a British colony. Wake up asshole, heroin is a major reason we're even here. It's Air America. The goddamn CIA's own war. We fly their goons, guns and drugs for them."

"Look around at everyone who's involved. Pull your head out of your ass."

My response? Fuck it. Where do I sign up?

My Insane Rage Drove Me to Join a CIA Assassination Team

By this point, my experiences in such a lunatic world of death and destruction had driven me into the depths of insanity. I felt the maniacal urge to go on the offensive.

In reality, I'd come to hate myself and wanted to die, but suicide was a cop-out.

My ideal solution was to join these covert Special Operations Group (SOG) missions, which were made up of CIA agents, Army Special Forces troops and Marines. Command control came from well-paid civilian CIA leadership with all active-duty military men participating in SOG missions considered volunteers on temporary loan. Any military man lost on covert duty simply got listed as missing in action.

No details about any death ever got released.

Gun support for the missions was coming from our Huey gunships. Painted distinctly white, the Air America aircraft that were participating in the operation would bring munitions to the anti-Communist war lords in the "Golden Triangle" – the corners of Laos, Burma, and Thailand. They would return loaded with heroin, a major cash crop worth millions of dollars, with portions of the black money used to fund the CIA's covert operations that also enriched corrupt local government and military leaders, along with the multi-national drug traffickers. All of the complex operations seemed like a win-win for those who were benefiting from it – a network that stretched across the world. Officially, as people were told, the heroin we saw being transported had been confiscated and got dumped into the ocean. Everyone suspected that was bullshit.

During the time I was in-country, these U.S.-sponsored covert operations had been expanding. Around our bases, the word spread that the CIA was actively seeking recruits to carry out their growing number of missions, involving hundreds of clandestine operatives and thousands of civilian targets.

"I'm in," I told them when invited.

One of SOG's active projects was associated with Operation Phoenix. We were utilizing psychological warfare tactics to demoralize civilian populations and reduce their support of the Viet Cong fighters. One of the most highly effective methods was to assassinate family members of local leaders and enemy sympathizers. That's what our team was directed to do.

By some administrative foul-up, I was never sworn to secrecy.

Crazed Killers – Mechanical and Unfeeling

Usually, assassination teams consist of insane but highly competent men. It's well known that men subjected to heavy combat for protracted periods of time crack up. Some become gun-shy and retreat into a passive, almost catatonic state of apathy, staring vacantly into space as solitary inhabitants of their world of pain. Others take on an offensive posture, losing all of the inhibitions of a normal human being in regard to killing another. Such warriors had become mechanical and unfeeling. It was from the ranks of these battle-induced psychotics that SOG assassination teams got filled.

I was one of them.

My team consisted of five guys: one civilian team leader, two Army Special Forces men, one Navy Seal, and myself. At our first meeting, in a hootch at Phu Bai, every member of the team looked and acted like a schizophrenic. We sat in the center of the dimly lit room on ammo boxes, two peeling and eating apples with their survival knives. With ordinary combat troopers, small talk always centered on women and food. With this group, the conversation turned on the relative potency of different hand-held weapons.

One guy regaled us with the virtues of the axe. He described an incident in which he pulled a single-handed surprise ambush on two gooks on patrol by dropping between them from a tree. Giggling with pride, he claimed that he so shocked them both that, before they could react, he had buried his axe in the face of one and shot the other in the gut with his pistol.

All of us listeners responded to his blusterous regaling with nervous laughter.

Strictly Civilian Targets

Since our operations were defined as strictly civilian, our military ranks meant nothing. Our team leader – we never knew his name – had served two tours in Vietnam as an Army Special Forces master sergeant and had now returned in-country as a CIA contractor. A short, stocky man who always looked unkempt, he had dark redbrown hair and the stubble of a beard on his face. When he looked at me with his beady brown eyes, it felt as if he was staring straight through me.

Behind his blank and affectless expression resided raw malevolence. Just being in his presence, I could feel the intense rage and hostility of this obviously cunning and adroit killer. In civilian life I would have considered him a dangerous paranoid schizophrenic and avoided any interaction with him.

Here, however, near the DMZ and after seeing so many dead and wounded, I felt comfortable with him as the leader of our assassination team. The other two members of our group – big, husky young kids who'd flipped out in combat – didn't radiate the wry cunning of savvy but certainly were savage fighters. Neither our leader nor I relied on these guys for anything other than covering our tails while we performed the tasks at hand.

Quiet Killings

With all volunteers already fully experienced in combat, we required little, if any training. We wanted to kill quietly. We preferred knives and garrotes. What instruction we got took place in that hootch at Phu Bai. Our Marine training made us adept at knife fighting.

We learned how to use the garrote from the civilian CIA men, our on-site instructors. Our unnamed lead instructor was a man in his late thirties with a solid build, he had dusty blond hair, bloodshot blue eyes, teeth yellowed by years of cigarette smoking, and the raspy voice of an alcoholic. His specialty was close-in assassination.

Working with a dummy, he showed us how to use the garrote – a thirty-inch length of metal aircraft throttle cable with metal dowels at each end to serve as handles. If we could get a position behind our prey, he assured us, the weapon was sure and silent. Once we slipped the cable over a victim's head, we could quickly chop with a scissors-like movement with our crossed arms.

"Make like you're punching with both fists," he explained. "You can kill anybody with this weapon if you use it right. Even a guy with a big bull neck will go down if you use the right motion. Make like you're hitting him from the back with short right and left crosses at the same time. Hit him and run. Don't wait around. If you do it right, the guy's dead right away. You'll know he's dead. There's no mistaking it. You'll know."

He never told us how we'd know.

This entire operation was strictly non-military – its planning, execution, and command lay totally out of the hands of the military. It was completely controlled by the CIA, which, as often opposed to the American military, was run by competent, dedicated men who took their projects seriously and planned them with great care, developing operations with exquisite precision.

Our team had carefully reconnoitered their operations and knew the details of topography and enemy strengths. Generally, we executed our missions flawlessly. The CIA may well have been made up of misguided patriots, brutes, or fanatics – but they definitely were not incompetent or cowardly.

Create The Diversion Then Strike the Home

The object of a typical mission consisted of creating a diversionary action around the edge of a village to draw the chieftain and his elders out of their hootches and into the fray. We created this with orbiting gunships that sprayed tracers and dropped loud explosive devices to set up a tremendous cacophony.

At the crescendo of this confusion, a CH-46A helicopter would drop into the village near the chieftain's hootch with a special assassination team that would run into the targeted residence and kill who was there.

Rather than have to eliminate enemy combatants, our grisly assaults on civilians were meant to dissuade any potential recruits or communist supporters by terrorizing and completely demoralizing their communities.

Our first hit was a Viet Cong stronghold, a little village about thirty miles southwest of Phu Bai. The CIA team carefully briefed us on the topography of the village, the stages of the operation, and emergency procedures. We set out at midnight – a flight of four Huey gunships and one CH-46A chopper, with no chase plane.

If we went down, that was it.

We flew in close formation guided by the tiny navigation lights on the choppers. After twenty-five minutes or so of flying, someone on the ground popped a yellow flare at which all of the choppers formed up in an orbiting circle. Then all hell broke loose as the choppers sprayed the ground with tracers and rockets. Looking down at the little village with its thatched-roof shelters, I could make out people scurrying around.

Then a spotlight from one of the Hueys briefly shone on a single hootch. The light flashed on, then off. That was our signal. We crash landed with the aft hatch of our chopper opening before the chopper actually touched down. Rapidly, the four of us jumped out of the back and ran toward the home the light had spotted for us. Once inside, in minutes, we had accomplished our gruesome directive, leaving the hootch littered with disfigured bodies and smeared with blood.

During the war, these covert missions were well-known and widespread.

Throughout the program, Operation Phoenix reportedly "neutralized" 81,740 people who were suspected of VC affiliation, of whom 26,369 were killed. Of those, 3,428 were assassinated.

Over a period of about four months, from October 1967 to January of 1968, I volunteered for these not-so-secret assignments. They'd call and I'd go. More often than not, our missions got aborted and we never touched down into a village – because the natives didn't fall in our trap and react how we wanted. Five of the missions I participated in, though, did go through – each time the details differed a little, but each time I killed people with my bare hands. Our debriefers kept assuring us of the enormous success of these kinds of missions – that they dealt a great psychological blow to our enemies.

We helping to win their war. Right?

Had we simply killed the chief outright, he would have become a martyr and his compatriots would have fought with renewed vigor. Since the villagers depended upon their leader for protection, his inability to defend his own family undermined their faith and confidence in him. Since the chief remained physically alive and well, he could not be deposed. This created massive unrest, distrust, disorganization and disillusionment among the local inhabitants, weakening the enemy's influence over them.

That's what our CIA debriefers told us. Is this our twisted approach to justifying our actions?

Close Call with Certain Death

On one of the other assassination missions, our rendezvous took place in that same hootch in Phu Bai with the same leader. This time our target was a village used at night for staging Viet Cong raids. As before, we planned to attack the chieftain's hootch shortly after sundown. We briefed carefully for the operation, plotted all of the coordinates, established all of our signals, and agreed on each man's role once we engaged our target. We studied the maps and determined our escape routes. If we had problems, we would escape to the rice paddies, then swim and crawl about five miles to the east, down a valley to a rise where the rescue choppers could recover us. We each always carried colored smoke grenades to identify our positions during a rescue operation.

Our plan was the same. Arriving at the village, the Hueys would lay down a diversionary barrage during which a CH-46A would drop us in. There, once dismounted, we would run for the chieftain's hootch, our leader with me right behind, while three young Navy Seals covered us outside. Once again, our job entailed killing that hootch's inhabitants, making as little commotion and noise as possible, and then returning to the waiting chopper.

Everything progressed smoothly until we landed in the village. The aft door of the chopper opened, and the five of us raced toward the hootch. Our leader charged up the stairs as I followed a few steps behind. The three Navy guys took up their positions at the entrance.

Our leader broke through the door and flashed his light around inside. I came up behind. "Nobody's here, Doc. Something's wrong!" he hollered.

Just then, I heard automatic weapons open up at the base of the hootch and looked back to see one of the Navy boys hit the ground in a pool of blood. A couple of rounds hit him square in the face, demolishing his head. The other two guys had started sprinting for the chopper.

"Come on! The gooks are here!" I hollered as I bolted back down the stairs toward the chopper. I could hear him in hot pursuit, his boots pounding down the stairs and the speedy cadence of footsteps in a dead run just behind me.

Then, all hell broke loose. Automatic weapon rounds sprayed from at least two positions at our rear. They were gunning for the chopper, with several rounds hitting its aft section, puncturing a fuel cell and hitting the left landing gear. Hurriedly, the crew chief started raising the aft ramp as the two remaining Navy guys vaulted over it while it rose, just as the bird prepared to take off.

I was too far behind so I cut off to the left, heading for the cover of a large rice paddy. While all the fire concentrated on the chopper as it took off, I dived and landed with a belly flop in foot-deep water. The furor aimed at the exiting chopper allowed me to hide myself among the high fronds of the rice plants that surrounded me. Aiding the 46 in its escape, the Hueys returned to spray the gooks, keeping them at bay.

Less than five minutes had transpired.

With night falling, the choppers had to break off. I knew they wanted to stay, but there was just no way they could come in to pick us up without being shot out of the sky. Besides, they had no idea where I was. I wondered whether our leader had survived and was also hidden somewhere under cover. Had I popped a smoke to identify my location, the gooks would have been on me much faster than our choppers. Our guys left with the hope we were still alive and, as planned, would be able to make it to the rescue zone for a pickup the following morning.

As the choppers flew off to the east, things quieted down, the sound of gunfire ceased. I stopped crawling, in case the gooks could see the motion in the paddy and identify my position. There I lay, flat on my belly, holding my head up, just out of the fetid paddy water. The gooks and their water buffalo had both shit in that water for fertilizer, so it smelled like a never-flushed toilet.

I froze still. After a few minutes I could hear the gooks sloshing through the paddy, looking for us. They suspected we'd been left behind and had set up a search to find us. For more than an hour, I could hear them tromping back and forth through the rice fronds, occasionally shouting to one another. Then as it became pitch dark, the sounds of footsteps quieted, leaving me alone – all alone, on my belly, in that cesspool. I didn't move a muscle for hours.

Goddamn, I'm scared.

The gooks must've been clued in. We were set up for an ambush.

I suppose I should be angry, but who are the good guys here?

And the bad?

If they find us, they'd furiously exercise their right to string us up in the center of the village.

After all, we came here to kill them.

Hours passed, with me frozen still as a statue, on my belly with my neck and shoulder muscles straining to keep my head out of that water. I couldn't sit up. If I did, they'd find me. If I relaxed and let my head down, I'd drown.

Damn. I'm thirsty.

207

Do I drink this shit-water?

Grimacing, I dipped my face into that vile fluid and allowed a few drops to penetrate my pursed lips. Initially, my stomach seized in an attempt to protect itself from the toxic liquid. Quietly, I began to gag. Then my stomach somewhat settled and I didn't puke what few drops I ingested.

I felt a bit of relief.

More hours crept along.

Guess I better start thinking about getting to the rescue zone.

It must be about three, and the choppers will be there around sunrise.

Crawling and walking took me just over an hour, which left me with a couple of hours to wait before any pick-up. I was really parched. I crossed a small stream whose water tasted much better. I rinsed my mouth and spat out the remnants of the foulness of my previous desperate attempts at hydration.

Hell, wish I'd brought Listerine or Chlorettes. Damn sure no kisses tonight.

Shut up, you sloppy shitface!

You are never leaving here alive.

As I hid near the rescue zone, I anxiously scanned the eastern sky for the choppers. Then I saw them, three dots above the horizon. I was thrilled, but silently celebrated. Our birds were flying at treetop level. As they approached, I could make out two Hueys and one CH-46A. When they had come to within about a mile or so of me, I popped my yellow smoke, which allowed them to establish an orbit over my position.

As I ran to the CH-46, I was given help by the gunner who had leaned out and grabbed me by the scruff of my neck and the back of my fatigues. I partly crawled and was further dragged aboard over the aft ramp. As the chopper lifted off the rise and into the sky, I fell face down onto the floor. I was soaking wet and chilled to the bone. I was shaking but smiling.

The crew chief was expectedly pleasant.

"Man, you smell like shit!" the gunner shouted.

"Yeah, and I feel like shit, too," I assured him.

"Where's our leader?" I shouted to the crew chief over the din. He

208

shrugged his shoulders and shook his head as if to say he didn't know.

"Ask the pilot if anybody's heard from him," I shouted. The crew chief gave me the thumbs up and started talking on the intercom.

"Nobody's seen him yet. Yours was the only smoke in the area. We'll go back in another couple of hours and pick him up. Maybe he'll walk back. Anyway, we'll get him back," he yelled into my ear.

No one ever saw him again.

We Tolerate Even Condone What We Do

In war, innocent people die. When our allies or friends are mistakenly killed by us, we exhibit remorsefulness and even pay money damages to survivors. When innocent civilians are assassinated, many consider that to be war crimes.

Even if they are, everyone seems to, at times, condone or at least tolerate them.

On March 16, 1968, in My Lai, thought to be a stronghold of the National Liberations Front, Charlie Company of the 11th Brigade was on a search and destroy mission, hunting for VC guerrillas, when a massacre occurred. By the time it ended, an estimated 504 civilians were dead, including 182 women, 17 of them pregnant, and 173 children. 56 of those were infants.

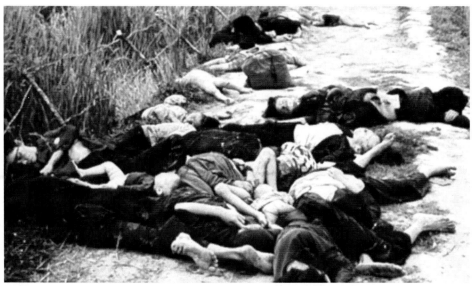

Photo taken March 16, 1968 by U.S. Army photographer. Laying motionless on the ground are My Lai villagers killed in the massacre (Source: U.S. Army, Ronald L. Haeberle)

At the time, morale was plummeting among U.S. soldiers, especially in the wake of the Tet Offensive, where Charlie Company had lost some 28 of its members to death or injury and had been reduced to just over 100 men.

Not a single shot was fired by an enemy combatant. They weren't there.

Huts were set on fire and anyone trying to escape was gunned down. Mothers were shielding their children when they were all shot. Young women were raped and mutilated. Countless livestock were slaughtered. One soldier later told a reporter, "I saw them shoot an M-79 (grenade launcher) into a group of people who were still alive. But it was mostly done with a machine gun. We met no resistance. It was just like any other Vietnamese village – old papa-sans, women and kids. I don't remember seeing (any) military-age male, dead or alive."

The U.S. military tried to cover it up, of course, but news finally broke – although it took 8 months for that to happen. Following the international outrage, the Army charged 14 men. All were acquitted except for Capt. William Calley, who many saw as a scapegoat. Calley was given a life sentence that was reduced to 20 years, and then to ten. He was paroled in 1974, three years after his conviction.

Later investigations revealed that Mi Lai was not isolated. A notorious U.S. military operation in the Mekong Delta called Speedy Express reportedly killed thousands of Vietnamese civilians and earned the commander of the operation the nickname "the Butcher of the Delta" for his principal role in the operation.

And during this war, as I can personally attest, the CIA assassinated civilian communist sympathizers and their families. All were considered our enemies.

We are horrified by stories of savagery we read about in conflicts across the world. But really? Is America not responsible for a history of war crimes? Is it hypocritical for us to condemn them, when we seem to tolerate them?

In his essay, *Should We Have War Crimes Trials?* by Neil Sheehan, first published in the New York Times on March 28, 1971, he writes: "The more perspective we gain on our behavior, the uglier our conduct appears. When the problem was held up to us, we paid no heed. We are finding out that we may have taken life, not merely as cruel and stubborn warriors, but as criminals. We are conditioned as a nation to believe that our enemies commit war crimes. The enemy's war crimes, however, will not wash us clean."

As this proxy war was, it was muddy and murky.

Chapter Twelve
Hated and Isolated at Home

"Society as a whole was certainly unable and unwilling to receive these men with the support and understanding they needed. The most common experiences of rejection were not explicit acts of hostility but quieter, sometimes more devastating forms of withdrawal, suspicion and indifference."
Christian G. Appy
Working Class War: American Soldiers and Vietnam
1993

I never thought I'd make it home. At the time, I didn't really care. However, the date came: February 3, 1968. My rotation date to depart for the United States. I had, in my grubby and encrusted hands, a pass home. I never imagined this time would come. I never expected it to happen.

Now, I didn't want to survive.

I can't get out of here alive.

I'm not sure who I am anymore.

Return to a "civilized" world?

How?

Pam's a hippie now. Make love not war.

Does she even want me?

Maybe I'll still get my chance to die.

A fallen hero, right?

I'm not gone yet.

Launch of the Tet Offensive

We'd heard about the enemy build-up with the Tet Lunar New Year approaching. For months, our battles along the DMZ had been escalating, in terms of frequency and scale as well as manpower and weaponry. Rocket attacks were raining down on Danang and Marble Mountain further to the south and the numbers of killed, missing or

213

wounded continued to mount by the tens of thousands. Attacks by sappers at our base's perimeters came to constitute a daily deadly threat.

"The longer the struggle lasts, the more your enemy's position deteriorates, both diplomatically and psychologically. Time is on your side, not the side of the imperialists."
Mao Tse-tung
Chairman, People's Republic of China

On January 31, 1968, days before my official release date, I was operating out of the Hue/Phu Bai base when the massive Tet Offensive was launched against us on multiple fronts. It spanned across South Vietnam including 34 of the 36 provincial capitals, 5 of the 6 largest cities, 50 hamlets and 23 military bases and airfields.

We'd been on a routine Medevac mission to Danang and had decided to stay overnight at Marble Mountain.

All Hell Broke Out Everywhere Simultaneously

That night, we were awakened by the deafening roar of what sounded like a freight train driving through the compound. Initially, I couldn't believe my ears. There wasn't a train for miles, and yet, that's was what I thought I heard. Then with a bright flash of light and a huge explosion, the entire compound shook and rumbled like an earthquake. I knew what was happening. We were under a rocket attack.

Incoming!
Another freight train, *BOOM!*
Then, *BOOM!*
Without even thinking, I ran for the bunker and hit the ground face down, with my helmet, flak jacket, M-14, and Unit 1.
Wow, they keep coming.
BOOM!
No kidding around here. We're getting hit really… really hard.
BOOM!
Holy shit.
The world is coming to an end.
I really ain't going to make it.
BOOM!
It's over.

214

In order to survive the concussion and shrapnel from close hits, we huddled down in our holes, face down in the dirt with our hands over our ears. All we could do was lie there, terrified.

No going anywhere – would our re-enforced structures protect us? Could they withstand a direct hit? Survival seemed to be by pure random luck. Trapped during what seemed like an eternity, we were being driven towards madness. Each hit and tremendous rumble would cause my spine to vibrate and my head to swim.

When it was over, an eerie silence hung in the air. Within minutes, the troops began to emerge, climbing out of their bunkers to assess the damage. Grim discoveries were made – a direct hit to a hootch with dead men inside who may have blown to pieces or others who looked like they were asleep, without a scratch on them, who'd been killed by the concussive forces alone.

Lost a Flight Surgeon Last Night

That next morning, we're all terribly anxious. We knew shit had just hit the fan. I felt depressed and strangely empty. I didn't really know why. As I sat at a table with Ron Reed, Curt Bohnan, and Art Lochridge, Lt. Col. Meyers, who sat at an adjacent table, had a grimace on his face, when he looked over at us. "Lost one of your guys last night, huh?"

"What do you mean?" I asked. Ron turned to me with a frown. "Down at Chu Lai, they also took some direct hits. Lost some guys, one of the flight surgeons was killed."

I bolted upright, my eyes widening. "Which one?"

There were three flight surgeons at Chu Lai – Frank Curran, Bill Dooley, and Stan Lewis – all of them were my close friends. I first met Frank and his wife through Class 112. Frank was a big, tall, strapping athletic fellow with sandy blond hair and blue eyes. A brilliant guy who had been an undergraduate philosophy major, he tended to be outspoken about his beliefs. He had received his medical degree from Cornell and completed an internship at New York's Bellevue Hospital. Frank had wanted to go into a psychiatry residency, but he became a victim of the 1965 Doctor's Draft and reluctantly joined the Navy. I never knew exactly how he got into the flight surgeon class, but he probably just enjoyed flying like the rest of us.

Highly vocal anti-war types, Frank and his wife shared many of my feelings about this rotten war. We hated it and constantly criticized the United States government. Such a vocal anti-war position probably made the Navy high brass happy to also send him to Vietnam. Since he wasn't one of their types, he was expendable like me. But I didn't want to see him go.

Bill Dooley was a happy-go-lucky Irishman who loved his booze. We were a lot alike. We'd been classmates at Illinois, and from those days on, I'd always known him as laughing and joking, who took medicine very seriously but loved to party. Like me, Bill was a smart, tough little guy who was from a poor Chicago working-class family. He'd also worked odd jobs through college and medical school, and always enjoyed cooking.

Although a fine doctor, like myself, Bill was also a lousy politician, shipped off to Southeast Asia. When we first started flight school, Bill was engaged to be married to Molly, an attractive dainty brunette who we all knew was the brains of the family. After learning that Bill wasn't going to avoid being shipped to Vietnam, she demanded they be married before he left. And married they were, with full military honors.

Bill was a good guy, a good doctor. I didn't want to lose him.

And Stan Lewis? All through the heaviest combat, I was comforted by the fact that there was someone who could take care of my beloved Pam if I didn't survive. Stan had specifically chosen Chu Lai with a fixed-wing fighter attack squadron, which was the one of the safest flight surgeon billets in-country. No Medevac activity came out of Chu Lai and there was no room for the flight surgeon in the fighter planes, so his only flying was on non-combat resupply missions. The last time I'd seen Stan, about two months earlier, he hadn't wanted to talk. Reserved and pale, I sensed his fear, as if he knew something was going to happen. I didn't want Stan to be the one. Stan couldn't die. I couldn't afford to lose him.

I didn't want to lose any of them, not any of them. I got up rapidly and asked again, "Don't you know which one it was? Which squadron was he with? His name?" The colonel shook his head as he bent it over a cup of coffee into which he peered. "Sorry, I just don't know. Why don't you give them a call?"

We all ran to the operations hootch, where I got on the phone, called down to Chu Lai and asked for the dispensary. Its phone rang. "Chu Lai Dispensary, HM-3 Sturgis speaking, sir."

"This is Dr. Levin at Marble Mountain. We heard you lost a flight surgeon last night. Who was it?"

"Dr. Lewis, sir." The words went directly to my gut. I doubled over. My face blanched. I didn't want to believe it was true.

Why wasn't it me!

I don't want Stan to be dead.

Anybody but Stan.

Not Stan, I don't want him dead.

On the phone, I was screaming in disbelief. "What happened?"

"Direct hit on the bunker. Three of them died."

"Can I talk to Dooley?"

"Yes sir, Dooley's here. Dr. Dooley's here."

A few moments of phone silence passed. I was quietly groaning and panting.

"Dooley here."

"Yeah, Bill, it's Al. What happened?"

"Well, Al, we lost Stan." Bill's voice was sober and tearful.

"What happened, Bill?"

"Direct hit on the bunker roof. The shell didn't penetrate. It exploded on the roof. I identified him. Not a mark on his body. Not a drop of blood anywhere. Must have been the concussion. Crushed his brains into hamburger..." his voice trailing off.

"Okay, Bill, thanks. Bye."

I'm nauseated.

Stan's dead.

Killed on the first day of the Tet offensive.

And I'm gonna make it back alive!

Descending Into Oblivion

I couldn't think. I couldn't talk. I just hurt. Inside, I was screaming.

No.

Not Stan.

It was supposed to be me.

I kept telling myself over and over – Stan was my reincarnation. After I got killed, he was going to go home and marry my widow and become a world-famous medical researcher. They would live happily ever after and would always remember me fondly, always remember me as I had once been – the big, strong, happy kid. They would always remember me smiling and laughing – as I wanted to be remembered. Because of them, I would never be forgotten. Now Stan was dead and I was still alive. He, the brilliant, gentle scientist, was gone.

I, who've tasted blood and can never again live as a civil human being, am alive.

I, the bitter, cynical killer, the surly, hollow-faced assassin, am alive.

For a week, I existed in a state of shock, sleepless hours filled with rageful outbursts and uncontrollable weeping. All I knew is that I was not heading home right away. Due to the Tet Offensive, my rotation to the States had been delayed. I was being forced back into duty, ordered to return to Hue/Phu Bai, to the University of Hue Hospital, being used by the U.S. military to treat the sudden spike in wounded soldiers and civilians due to the huge escalation in the war.

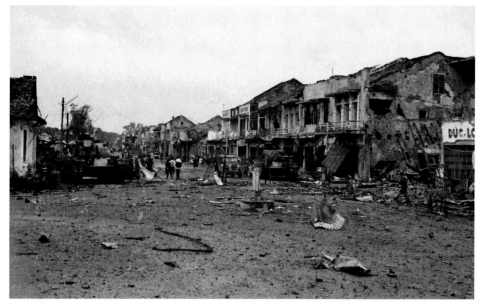

Damage from Battle for Hue during Tet Offensive (Source: USMC)

Hospitals near heavy action were under constant red alerts with the staff wearing flak jackets and helmets. During attacks, patients were shoved under their beds and mattresses thrown over them for protection. When the power was out, the staff performed mouth to mouth or mouth to trach breathing for the wounded on respirators or with chest tubes. Not all lived to see the electricity restored.

While I was nearly paralyzed mentally and emotionally, I was greatly relieved to be working in an actual hospital setting, away from any combat, on patients already triaged and not in the throes of death. Tormented by a crippling psychic pain, part of me hoped against hope that I would still be killed. Another perverse force though now welled up inside of me – an obstinate desire to go home, to dedicate the rest of my life to bettering the world.

I was still haunted by perseverating thoughts of suicide.

It would have been so easy – just to jump off a helicopter into a firefight. It would have been so quick – just keep my head up when the bullets were flying by. It would have been so madly exhilarating – just get up and walk around during an artillery barrage.

So easy.

Somehow, though, my primal survival instinct prevailed.

On February 12th, back at Marble Mountain, as the Tet Offensive continued to rage intensively across I Corps and elsewhere, I was preparing to return home, stumbling around the base trying to gather my wits enough to be able to just get out of the country. I was so severely depressed. I was still grieving deeply over the unexpected loss of my dearest of friends.

Can I even continue to breathe?

Can I even link one thought to another?

I was completely wasted.

Tet's Departing Gift

To get to Danang Air Base from Marble Mountain, we loaded up into a Jeep and drove. Somehow, I realized this would be the last time I'd ever make this journey, going over the river, past the wooden towers used as gun emplacements with the South Vietnamese ARVN soldiers and their automatic weapons trained on the crowds, watching very closely, looking to see if any gooks were going to throw grenades or start shooting.

We drove through Danang and up to the operations shack at the air base. Just as the door closed behind me, as I was about to tell them who I was and show them all of my baggage, it started again, all of a sudden, commencing with the roaring of sirens, after which the freight trains started arriving.

Whoosh, *BOOM!*

Whoosh, *BOOM!*

Those fuckers won't give up.

They want me dead.

Whoosh, *BOOM!*

Rockets, hitting us in Danang!

Goddamn it, I'm supposed to be getting out of here!

Here we are sitting with a C-130, ready to go. And, we're gonna get blown to pieces.

Whoosh, *BOOM!*

Terrorized, I hit the floor, face down, hands over my head.

Can't I just get the hell out of here?

I'm Out! Or Am I?

Everybody waited, poising themselves. Ten minutes or so had passed. Nothing. Then, I saw our flight crew run to the C-130 and start up the engines. Spontaneously, we also broke for the bird. There must have been fifty of us running helter-skelter, carrying our bags and our trunks, frantically loading the aircraft with all of our belongings, trying to get the hell out of the country before the next attack got underway.

The C-130's engines roared up as I sat back in my seat and locked myself into the seat belts. We started taxiing towards the active runway, accelerating faster and faster until we made it onto it. We didn't stop, just went to full engine speed on the take-off. After a few tense moments, we were airborne.

Am I finally out of this stinking country?

I'm gonna live?

Oh, no!

Out the window, I saw the left outboard engine sputtering, then stop.

Shit! We've lost an engine.

Sure, why not?

We still had three engines.

This bird can make it on three engines.

"Let's keep going! Get us the hell out of here!" I shouted toward the cockpit, as if the pilots could hear me.

Damn it, we're turning around in the pattern to land.

I guess that's smart. We have to go over the ocean to Okinawa.

If we lost more engines, we'd be in the drink.

After we made an uneventful landing back at Danang and taxied up to the operations shack, one the crew members came out of the cockpit. "I don't think it's anything serious, guys. I think we just popped a fuel line or something like that. Won't be more than ten or fifteen minutes. Don't unload. Stay aboard the airplane."

The maintenance crew rushed toward the aircraft, pulled the cowling from the engine and started working on it. Ten minutes or so later, they put the cowling back on again and gave the pilot the thumbs up. The crew then anxiously started running up the engines one more time.

Lord, maybe we're going to make it out this time!

With the engines churning, we started taxiing towards the active runway again, progressed onto our takeoff roll, and then were airborne, with all the engines churning.

Is it true? Are we going to make it out of here alive?

Holy shit! We're back in the air.

We're out over the ocean. We're safe!

Stopover in Okinawa

Could I actually start thinking about a tomorrow? A day not filled with mayhem and terror.

I could feel only an enormous hollowness in my chest and my gut. I'd left something behind in Vietnam. I'd left an idealistic, happy-go-lucky kid. He was dead and buried back there. The person returning home had the same name, but that's where the similarity ended. A year

221

earlier, I arrived in Vietnam, weighing a hundred eighty-five pounds – a big, strong jock, always smiling. I left there 45 pounds lighter, gaunt and haggard, with hollow cheeks and dark, sunken eyes. I was now a killer, a bitter, cynical and depressed U.S.-sponsored covert assassin.

It's not exactly uplifting chatter around the water cooler or family dinner table.

The flight to Okinawa might have lasted three or four hours – I don't even know. All I know is I spent it in a daze, unable to fathom exactly what was going to happen to me, not equipped to handle anything that was going to befall me in the future. I could deal with combat. I could deal with the horribly mutilated young men and the primitive medical facilities. I could deal with rocket and mortar attacks. I could deal with small arms fire. I could even deal with getting shot down in a helicopter. But I couldn't conceive of how to deal with being at home.

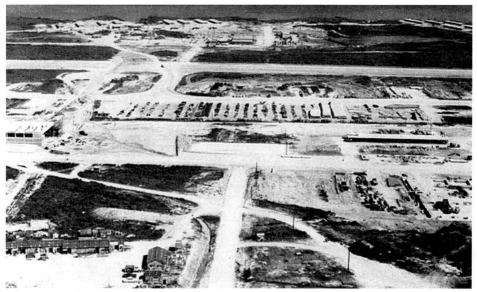

Aerial view of U.S. Marine Corps Station Okinawa (Source: USMC)

I didn't know how I would react.

We arrived in Okinawa at about four in the afternoon and were scheduled to take off at nine the next morning aboard a Pan Am 707 that would fly us into Travis Air Force Base in California. The C-130 that had brought us to Okinawa came from the squadron whose flight

222

surgeon was Bill Fowler, a nice, quiet guy from Oklahoma. He had been in general practice when he too got trapped by the Doctor's Draft and we'd been in the same flight surgeon class.

Bill lucked out by getting a billet in Okinawa with the C-130 squadron. Like all of the other transport-associated aviation personnel, he saw only a minimum of combat, and that only for short periods of time. I got to Bill's hootch and decided to spend the night with him, sharing about Stan's death. He'd expected it. We'd already lost a number of our classmates, and to Bill, Stan would just be one more. I don't know exactly how I told Bill about Stan. I know that I couldn't stop bursting into tears every time I thought about it. Stan had been a close friend. Stan had been me. Bill understood. Bill knew that Stan and I had been close. He was warm and comforting.

Finally U.S. Bound

After we had dinner that night, I hit the rack early for a few hours of sleep, still abruptly interrupted by constant nightmares, re-living my combat experiences and the grisly horrors I had experienced. Such nightly occurrences were often crippling.

In the morning, I boarded the Pan Am flight, strapping in for the long fourteen-hour ride from Okinawa to Travis Air Force Base. For me, probably like many others, this flight proved a surrealistic experience. Here I was sitting safely and quietly aboard a jet airplane, something that had become totally unfamiliar. The aircraft was clean, no one was going to shoot it down, and there were women aboard, who smiled and served us hot meals and beverages.

Maybe I did die and mistakenly got sent to heaven.

Captivated by my view out the window, I'd drift off to sleep, then awake to eat – but I don't really remember much of it. All I know is that I was totally unprepared. I'd expected to die. I wanted to. I never anticipated that I'd be actually aboard a civilian jetliner and homeward bound.

We stopped at Guam for refueling, I got out for a few minutes and went to the PX, where I bought a beautiful bottle of Napoleon brandy. I figured that I was going to buy the most expensive booze possible and get as drunk as I could as soon as I got home.

Following what seemed like forever, as the plane began its final approach, I remember seeing landfall – the lights of California from the air at about seven in the evening. I couldn't believe it. There it was, the Golden Coast. I still didn't think I would make it. I was sure we were going to crash and burn on landing. There was no way I could survive, no way I could live through that horrific tribulation. And then, the flaps came down and the landing gear did, too. We made a nice, soft, uneventful landing.

For the first time in thirteen months, I was on continental American soil, and I was alive. Against my fervent desire, I had survived the Vietnam war.

Touching Down at Home

After we taxied up to the ramp, we got herded off the airplane.

There must have been about a hundred and fifty of us who went through a perfunctory customs check. With that many, there were only two officials to check our luggage. They didn't give a shit, though. All they did was funnel us through large empty rooms cordoned off with ropes. They just pushed us along, like so many cattle. No smiles, no "welcome homes," just "move it, soldier." Then one guy, at the end of the line yelled, "The buses are over that way. The taxis are over here. Good-bye and good luck."

"Thanks for nuthin', asshole," one of the troopers from the planeload riposted.

What a hell of a way to come home! No bands. No flags waving. No nothing. Shit, I hoped I had a dime to call home. The assholes didn't even tell us where the goddamn phones were!

Finally, I found a pay phone, dialed up the house, called my wife and, after a year away, announced, "Honey, I'm at Travis."

"What? You're in the United States? What happened? How come you're back so soon?" were the first words uttered to me by my beloved wife.

"What do you mean, so soon? I was supposed to be back two weeks ago. The fuckin' Tet Offensive!" I exclaimed.

"Oh, I didn't mean it that way." She responded, "I mean, well, I called the Navy base and they told me you were extended for another month. This is such a surprise. Come on home. Take a cab."

Take a cab?

"Yeah, okay," I replied. "I'm just gonna hop into a cab and come home. How long do you think it'll be?"

"Oh, about forty-five minutes," she estimated.

"Okay, I'll be in a cab and be there in less than an hour." A bit perplexed, I picked up all of my luggage and climbed into a taxi. Little did I know that my phone call triggered the fastest moving job in Berkeley's sordid history. Her latest suitor was being freshly dispatched out of back door by a clan of her hippie friends, while my wife met me on the front stairs with a big kiss.

I was in ecstasy, at least for the moment.

Viewed As a Freak

For me, trying to adjust to the abrupt change from combat in Vietnam to Berkeley's hippie culture proved almost impossible. Everywhere I went, people viewed me as a freak. They would ridicule me for being so stupid for going to war. They treated me like scum, a second-class citizen. Pam, my own wife, would look at my emaciated body with revulsion and say in a fit of anger, "The Marine Corps makes mice!"

During my first week at home, I found it impossible to relax. I couldn't speak to anyone without breaking into tears. I paced the floors for hours reciting the names of all my dead friends. I awoke at night with shrieking nightmares. My greatest fear was that I would forget the names of my dead buddies. I felt I was the only living human that really cared about them. I couldn't forget them.

I couldn't interact. I wasn't cool. I was such a misfit that I caused Pam much embarrassment. Those first few days were horrible. I was immensely thankful to her for not throwing me out of the house that I was paying for.

Back on Duty

Upon returning from Vietnam, I was entitled to one month's leave, but since I had such difficulty in making the transition to civilian life, I decided to report to my next duty assignment, the Alameda

225

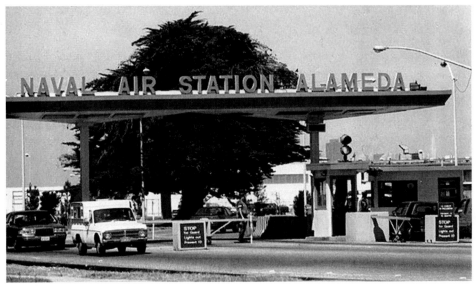

Front gate of Alameda Naval Air Station in California (Source: U.S. Domain)

Naval Air Station, three weeks early. It was far easier to relate to active-duty military personnel than to civilian citizens. I was still officially attached to the Marines, so my commanding officer was Colonel Smiley, an old Marine Corps fighter pilot.

Since I was a doctor, I was on loan to the Navy Medical Dispensary under the command of Captain Grenstein, a weird bird with an Irish Catholic mother and a Jewish father, who had walked out on the family when the captain was a child. From then on, the captain hated Jews. If that wasn't bad enough, he acted like Captain Queeg in *The Caine Mutiny*. He demanded rigid military discipline, sharp uniforms and snappy salutes. Needless to say, it didn't take long for us to butt heads.

I hadn't worn Navy uniforms for over a year, during which I had lost forty-five pounds. As a consequence, my uniforms drooped all over, including my hat. Since I had only four more months of obligated active duty to go, I saw no sense in getting them refitted. To add insult to injury, my black socks mysteriously disappeared, so I often wore argyles with my uniform. In full dress Navy blues I looked more like a refugee from a Salvation Army thrift store than a naval officer.

Beyond that, many of the enlisted medical corpsmen at the base were men with whom I had served in Vietnam, guys that I considered close friends. Despite the difference in our ranks, we were always on a first-name basis. This incensed the Captain and he vowed to make my last four months on active duty miserable.

Colonel Smiley liked me. Fully aware of what I had just gone through, he knew I was treading a razor thin line between sanity and schizophrenia. He took it upon himself to do whatever was reasonable to keep me sane until I could leave active duty. The Colonel knew of Captain Grenstein's feelings and tried his best to protect me from his wrath as much as possible. He rigged an assignment in which we were required to fly once a week in a Marine Corps airplane to Camp Pendleton, where I taught corpsmen about Medevac missions. During those trips, we conversed quite a bit. The Colonel, who'd come along to visit his son, a Marine captain, tried earnestly to ease my transition from combat to civilian life.

While at the base, I was scheduled to get some medals for my service in Vietnam. These included the Silver Star, the Bronze Star with Valor and Air Medals. Thinking it would be good public relations as well as helpful to my psyche to give me a formal ceremony, the base brass informed me I should invite my family and be at the grandstand at 0830 in the morning. I had no idea what was going to happen, so I complied. As it turned out, there was a parade, complete with marching band, for one person, me, and one spectator, my wife. The whole scene must have been ridiculous to watch. In any case, Captain Grenstein arrived at the dispensary at 0900 and promptly asked for me.

"Where the hell's Levin? He's late again, that fool."

"No sir, he's not late," one of the medical corpsmen on duty responded. "He's out there," and pointed to the parade grounds.

"You mean he's in that parade and he didn't invite me to the reviewing stand? I'm his commanding officer. He can't do that to me. That's bad conduct. He'll pay for this," Grenstein sputtered as he hurried out the door and down the street in order to be in the reviewing stand by the time I passed by. I remember seeing the old duffer sprint by me, still sputtering invectives from his puffy red face. He was going to get a salute out of me if it cost him a coronary! The medical corpsmen thought this was hysterical and whooped with laughter.

Such levity helped, for medical dispensary duty was awfully boring. All we basically ever did was give medications to active-duty personnel or take care of their dependents. The flight surgeons on the base spent a bulk of their time giving physicals to the aviation personnel. Our medical skills were hardly summoned, much less taxed as we performed exams, ordered labs, wrote scripts, stitched lacerations, lanced boils and performed circumcisions.

Before many of the Marines left for Vietnam, Alameda Naval Air Station was the final Stateside duty station. Hearing that Vietnam was absolutely filthy, many uncircumcised Marines chose to have the operation before going to war so as to prevent infection of the penile foreskin, known as balanitis, a common problem in combat. As I've described, while in combat, men don't get their pants off for days or even a week or more. Sometimes they are forced to urinate lying down, so they'd live in soiled underwear for extended periods of time.

While there, being pretty good at circumcisions, I was being called upon for my services, but since I had become clueless as to standard operating procedure, I paid no attention to the base's Flight Physical Schedule.

One morning, I had a circumcision scheduled while, unbeknownst to me, all the other flight surgeons were on leave. I was the only one there. As luck would have it, the captain had scheduled a flight physical for the admiral to start promptly at 0800. Well, as it turned out, I was a bit distracted at the time, operating on a guy a bit tense about having his penis cut on. My patient happened to be a twenty-three-year-old sergeant due to be shipped out in two months and quite nervous about the whole operating room scene. I had injected the Novocaine and started my first cut, when all of a sudden the operating room door flew open and in barged Captain Grenstein, in his street clothes.

"Levin, what the hell do you think you're doing?"

"I'm doing a circumcision under sterile conditions, so get the hell out of my operating room in your street clothes."

"This is the uniform of the United States Navy, and if you'll notice the insignia on my collar, I am a captain," the old man sputtered. "You are only a lieutenant. You cannot speak that way to a superior officer."

"I am a doctor and this is my patient so get the hell out. I'll talk to you later."

Grenstein was really steamed. Almost out of control, he turned around and stomped out of the room. This poor sergeant on the table had never heard such an exchange between two officers, which was especially disconcerting inasmuch as one of the two of the combatants was chopping on his private part! Thank goodness the rest of the operation proceeded without incident despite the fact that I was fuming at the old son of a bitch for barging into a sterile field without gowning up.

After the surgery I took off the scrub suit, donned my uniform, then charged down to the captain's office, where he bellowed at me. "I had the Admiral waiting for a flight physical while you did a goddamn circumcision!"

"I don't care who was waiting. You had no right to barge into the operating room and act like a perfect ass in front of a terrified patient," I hollered back. "You may be a military officer, but I'm a doctor and don't you ever forget that!"

Grenstein fumed, turned beet red and lost his cool. "Goddamn it Levin, I'm gonna get you. I'm gonna get you. I'm gonna drag you to the admiral's office myself. I'm gonna court-martial you. You're gonna spend the next two years in the brig, you can bet on that."

He grabbed at my tie. Because I was wearing a clip-on, it detached from my collar and fell limply into his fist. Still holding my cheap accessory, he grabbed my lapel with his other hand and hollered, "Come with me!" and charged out of the dispensary with me in tow.

By this time, I was too upset to appreciate the humor of the situation.

The air base is built like a college campus, with its administration buildings situated around a grassy court. The dispensary stood two buildings away from the admiral's office. Here we were, two commissioned officers, marching across the courtyard in tandem. I was furiously angry, just barely able to restrain myself from killing the little asshole dragging me by the lapel. Grenstein, red in the face and puffing with fury, angrily strutted. Everyone on the base by now knew of the discord between us. Everyone watched the scene amused. "There they go again!"

We finally barged into the office of the admiral, who had been forewarned but still had a hard time keeping a straight face. Grenstein started screaming at the top of his lungs about my insubordination and my miserable military bearing. The admiral tried, as best he could, to look serious, but it was all he could do to keep from bursting out in laughter. Finally, he found himself able to speak.

"Okay, Captain, why don't you leave? I'll take care of the Lieutenant myself."

That brought Grenstein back to his senses. He snapped a salute and left the room. The admiral looked me over carefully. Disheveled, I now had no tie and my coat was four sizes too big.

"Levin, you know you are in the Navy, and in our esteemed outfit you must obey the orders of senior officers. Just try to remember that until you get out, please."

"Yes sir." I found myself somewhat embarrassed about the ridiculous scene we had made. "I'm sorry, sir."

"Dismissed," the Admiral responded with a wink. Grenstein was also embarrassed, so we avoided one another for the next several weeks.

Extreme Difficulty Adjusting

Meanwhile, I was having real difficulty adjusting to civilian life. Bit by bit, I found it nearly impossible to carry on a conversation with an ordinary person without crying. My wife was exceedingly unhappy. Through no fault of her own, she found herself forced to live with an insane stranger, a man who couldn't even try to rest without a loaded rifle at his side. A man who frequently awoke from nightmares in a pool of sweat, screaming the names of dead men. A man nothing like the man she had fallen in love with and married. A man who constantly embarrassed her in front of her friends. A man who represented nothing but an obstacle between herself and true contentment.

I tried to integrate as a civilian, including taking several moonlighting doctor jobs to earn quick cash. I was scheduled to be released from active duty around June 15, 1968, but emancipation time came and went. With the excuse that he didn't have enough flight surgeons, Grenstein kept delaying my release. Then our final confrontation came. We were scheduled to perform an inspection at Leemore Naval Air Station in California's Central Valley. That meant that three flight surgeons were required to go to Leemore to inspect records, shoeshines, and latrines for the various squadrons. I was scheduled to be one of the three to go.

The diversion made me happy until I learned it would be a two-day deal and that we were to stay at the base overnight. That was the straw that broke the camel's back. I knew I could not spend one more night with the military, away from home, and remain sane. I knew I would crack. "Why don't I fly myself down to Leemore on the first day, then come back for the night and fly back the next day?" I suggested to Grenstein. "After all, I am a qualified pilot and there is no sense in my being on the base all night."

"Levin, you'll go with everyone else and spend the night there. I don't want to hear any more out of you."

"Captain, I cannot go away from home anymore. I cannot be sent away by the military anymore."

"You will go, and that's an order!" Grenstein bellowed.

"I'm sorry, sir. I won't go."

"You are refusing an order! That's the last straw. I'm going to have you court-martialed yet!" He shouted as he stormed off to his office. I quickly ran to a telephone and called Colonel Smiley. "Goddamn it, Levin, can't you ever stay out of trouble? By the way, when are you supposed to get out?"

"Any time now."

"Well, when do you want to get out?"

"How about last week, Colonel?"

"Today is your last day. Get ready to sign out." This was music to my ears. I was going to become a civilian! I was walking on air. Just then, Grenstein came steaming out of his office. Apparently the admiral had another solution.

"Levin, I just talked with the admiral. We decided either you're crazy or you're court-martialed. I'm sending you for an emergency psychiatric evaluation now!"

Acute Adult Situational Reaction

So off I went, dutifully, to bare my psyche to the base shrink, a career Navy commander. All he wanted to do was play golf. He seemed put off by having to deal with the likes of me. After I described the entire episode, he summarily wrote it off as an "Acute Adult Situational

Reaction" – whatever the hell that means.

Functionally, that meant that I was too crazy to be court-martialed but not crazy enough to receive a disability. So, the base inspection in the Central Valley went on with two flight surgeons, while I was required to man emergency call at the dispensary that night. At least I didn't have to go out of town.

Colonel Smiley had a good belly laugh at the diagnosis. "Levin, if we kept you around here any longer, you'd make a shambles of the entire base. I want you out of the service now. Start signing out right now."

When you sign out of the service, you go to the head of each department and get his approval to be released. Grenstein told me that he wanted to be the last on my list. When I finally got to him, I found him sitting behind his desk with a sardonic smile. "I've got to let you go for now, but don't get rid of your uniforms. I'm going to get you back into the Navy!" he glowered.

Find Me Under My Bed

I didn't respond, just shivered and handed him my papers. He signed, I saluted and left. After turning in the paperwork, I went straight home and told Pam what he had said, then calmly went upstairs to the bedroom. Several hours later she went looking for me and found me under the bed. I had brought along a pillow from the bed itself, my knife, and a book – then had laid down under the bed, curled up, and commenced reading.

"What are you doing?" Pam asked, incredulously.

"Just reading a book."

"But you're under the bed!"

"I'm hiding here because they're going to come after me."

"Who's coming after you?"

"The Navy wants me back."

"Oh." Student of psychology that she was, she was going along with my insanity. "But how about dinner? We're going to eat dinner now."

"Okay. Then bring it up here so nobody can find me." I believe that my tone sounded perfectly sane.

"Oh, of course, so nobody can find you," she replied as she backed to the door, returning shortly with my dinner. She was nice enough to bring up her own plate, too, and join me in the bedroom. I was totally psychotic, but feigning sanity.

During that entire evening, Pam tried to coax me out from under the bed. But I would come out only to go to the bathroom, then slip back under. That night, as she slept on the top of the bed, I slept under it with my knife at the ready. All that time, I thought I was acting sane. To me, what I was doing made perfect sense. Crazy as it was, obviously ridiculous as I see it now, I thought that as long as I was under the bed, nobody could find me. It must have been ludicrous to see a grown man hiding under the bed, but at the time it seemed the only way to stay out of continued military service.

Finally, after that day and night and the next full day and that night during which again Pam slept on top with me under that bed, she lost her patience. But in what probably represented her last act of kindness to me, in tears, she called my cousin Theresa, who lived nearby. "He's totally crazy. He's under the bed. He won't come out."

So Theresa and Bill, her husband, came over. They just sat there and talked to me. Bill was a psychiatric social worker who had been in the military and was now in the reserves, so he knew all about military service and how to talk to veterans. He assured me that the Navy really didn't want me any more than I wanted them, that it was totally irrational to think that they would want to call back such a crazy troublemaker.

After a while, they had me laughing. And following about an hour of talking, I came out from under the bed and went on with my life. But it took years for me to realize just how deranged I had been for those two days and nights.

Now I can say that the bed then was my protection from the world that started crashing down. Something was above me. That's what it was. It wasn't necessarily that I thought I was hidden, but somehow, the bed would shelter me from harm. At the time it seemed totally reasonable.

When the world starts disintegrating around you, you try to find safe shelter.

And that's what I did.

California Dreaming

When I got home from Vietnam, Pam shared that she wanted to remain in Berkeley, enjoying the lifestyle and social structure that it had become so famous for in the late sixties. So, I got on the phone and called Dr. Fred Rosen, my old boss at Harvard, described my situation, and asked whether I could continue my once budding career as an immunologist.

Yes, he assured me, I could do that – I should go to work with Dr. Hugh Fudenberg at the University of California in San Francisco, as Dr. Fudenberg was a noted expert in immunology and had an active and productive training program.

When I called Dr. Fudenberg, he told me that a slot was opening up that was ideal for me. On the day I began my postdoctoral training at UCSF, I was actually excited and eager to rehabilitate myself into the civilian world.

Unfortunately, UCSF was not ready for Vietnam veterans. At the time, the UCSF medical school was hungry for government and defense contractor funds to expand its research programs. They wanted to avoid even the appearance of any controversy. That included not having any Vietnam veterans working for them. In those days, we were sub-class citizens and certainly not eligible to be mingling among the elite of the academic medical establishment. I never wore anything other than short-sleeved shirts and cotton pants with moccasins – no underpants, so socks, no belt.

I was a freak to them, and they didn't want me.

Denied Typical Veteran Benefits

Through the Veterans Administration, I had applied for educational benefits, but was told by UCSF that I was ineligible. That opinion came from the administrator in charge of the program there.

A plump, proper-looking women in her mid-fifties sitting behind an unusually neat desk, Ms. Beatrice Carmon glanced up at me over her Ben Franklin half-glasses – perturbed at my interruption, looking like a no nonsense schoolteacher about to discipline the class troublemaker.

"What can I do for you?" she asked.

"My name is Alan Levin. I've just joined the postdoctoral fellowship program with Dr. Hugh Fudenberg, and I'd like to apply for veterans' benefits."

"You're already here and you're not registered with the Veterans Administration?" she asked incredulously.

"I guess so. I was told you could help me."

"All of the veterans come here with their applications already approved. You come in here asking for benefits, and I don't even know you're a veteran." With that, she pulled my record and reviewed it. Her face began to droop as if further disenchanted. "There is no record of your having served at all at the National Institutes of Health in any research or education programs. Is that correct?"

"Yes, that's true."

"Well, all you have done, according to this record, is go to Vietnam. Isn't that true?"

"Ma'am, all the other guys were at NIH. I was in Vietnam," I responded to her quiet hostility, barely able to keep my anger under control.

"Then what are you doing here? I'm not at all sure that Vietnam veterans are eligible for benefits at this institution. Your kind of benefits are for learning to be a car mechanic or something, aren't they?" accompanying this final query with a sly and sardonic smile as her bulky mass continued to solidly occupy her swivel chair. I just stood there stunned, disbelieving, unwilling to accept what I had just heard, then left.

Several days later, I recounted my experience to a new friend, Dr. Harold Varmus, who had come from the NIH at the same time that I had arrived home from the Vietnam war. Harold had comfortably served his military obligation in the virology labs and just like all of his fellow graduates, his VA benefits had been quickly approved. Sensitive and compassionate, Harold was outraged at what I told him and went to his boss, Dr. Michael Bishop, who was also sympathetic. After nine months of their constant prodding, the UCSF finally agreed that Vietnam veterans were indeed eligible. Those two colleagues, Drs. Varmus and Bishop were not only caring human beings, they were also incredibly gifted scientists, sharing the 1989 Nobel Prize in Medicine.

Pam And I Not Happy Ever After

As a young married couple, Pam and I wanted a lot of children. We couldn't conceive and decided to adopt a one. I was a physician, capable of earning a good living. With the money we had saved from my combat pay and what income I was able to earn by moonlighting in emergency rooms, we made a down payment on her dream house: a veritable mansion in Berkeley, with chauffeur's quarters over the garage and maid's quarters in the basement.

Using the skills I had learned working construction in earlier years, I upgraded both surplus units into nice little apartments with rental income covering our mortgage payment.

Our home established, we went to the Children's Home Society in Oakland. It might seem unusual to actually get a child to adopt as quickly as we did, but here was this young couple with difficulty bearing children. One was an R.N. and the other an M.D. What better adoptive parents could anyone imagine? The social worker quickly lined us up with a college student about to deliver a child that she wanted give up for adoption.

Pam and I never met the parents, but we got Eric when he was a newborn.

Within two months after we had adopted this child, my wife informed me that she would have preferred that I had died in Vietnam, that the person she knew had. When it came to dealing with civilian life, I suffered such a low self-image that I simply complied and left, moving into a one-room apartment.

Within less than month, Pam phoned me – she hadn't realized how much trouble it was to raise an infant. She was calling me to pick up Eric – or she would return him. Dutifully, I responded and moved the child into my one-room apartment. So, I became a single father, caring for a baby in a one-room apartment and doing medical research.

I slept on a hide-a-bed in the main room and Eric slept in the walk-in closet. There I was, changing diapers and feeding a three-month-old while completing a full postgraduate program in clinical immunology. It could've been a lot worse than it was. Living nearby was a Mexican family that was more than happy to care for Eric while I worked. Any girlfriend I had needed to possess maternal instincts and tolerate this quirky single father with a Dodge station wagon, loaded with the playpen in the back and a kid's hand prints all over the rear window!

Although I was working in pediatrics at the hospital with my tiny apartment nearby, I was an ill-prepared parent. All I knew was that I had to feed, clothe, and protect the child. I perceived my sole obligation to him was to keep him alive. I knew absolutely nothing about nurturing or affection. I was in such bad shape myself that I was unable to bond with my son.

Then, unexpectedly, Pam called to inform me that she had married, settled down, and was ready to raise our child. I brought him to her. I've seen him just twice in the ensuing years. Thankfully, Eric had a family with a normal life, so much better than what I was providing for him.

Prior to Vietnam, Pam and I earned more money than we'd ever had before, enjoyed more free time than ever before, lived in perfect weather, and worked at dream jobs. Then, slowly, another reality sank in – the war. Our friends were being wounded, killed, and widowed.

Then I got drafted and shipped out.

Pam knew where I was. She watched in horror the battles in TV news footage the day after it happened, while it always took at least ten days for my letters to arrive. She never knew whether I was alive or dead. So, the safest way to keep her sanity was to fall out of love with me.

I can't blame her for that. When I returned, I was a different person, certainly not the man she had married. She didn't like the new me. I understand. I didn't like the new me either. Why saddle a young woman looking into a bright future with a strange man she doesn't want?

Had it not been for Vietnam, we would still be married today – perhaps adopting other kids – me as a professor at Harvard or Stanford.

Who knows?

The IRS Is After You

Around this time, I received notice that I was to be audited by the

Internal Revenue Service – for the year I'd spent in Vietnam. During the audit, I learned that the Navy had paid the Marine Corps $35 a month for my room and board on a temporary additional duty assignment. This $35 a month for the bulk of the year 1967 represented the expenses for a hole in the ground, sandbags, and C-rations. It turned out that the IRS considered this payment as ordinary income and penalized me for not reporting it as such.

I was outraged by this harassment. I hated my government. Then came what I considered the crowning blow when the postman delivered a box to me. It contained a brand-new London Fog raincoat my folks had bought at Lyttons in Chicago, some of my favorite cheeses, a newsy letter from my mother, and an official package addressed to me from the Department of the Navy, dated September of 1968. Since I had never provided a permanent address, the Navy only had that of my parents in Skokie to use in sending anything to me.

First, I pulled out the raincoat. Mom knew I liked the Ivy League look and she was trying to lift my spirits. Yet it didn't quite work out like that. When I proudly donned the coat, the sleeves hung long and the shoulders drooped. I looked in the full-length mirror on my closet door. The coat appeared enormous. What a disappointment. They had sent the wrong size. Then, I looked at the tag: 42 Long.

That's my size. Why doesn't it fit?

Then it dawned on me.

I used to be a hundred eighty-five pounds.

I was feeling fit as a fiddle – like the song.

"Fit as a fiddle and ready for love, I could jump over the moon up above, Fit as a fiddle and ready for love, Haven't a worry, I haven't a care, Feel like a feather that's floating on air."

Al Goodheart/Al Hoffman/Arthur Freed

Now, in the mirror, I was peering at the withered frame of a man now long gone. Defeated, I took off the coat, laid it down on a chair and sobbed.

Piss On My Silver Star

After a brief time, I became curious about the Navy package, which I opened to discover a fancy official-looking box, a blue rectangular container with gold filigree around its sides. On the top was

238

inscribed "Silver Star." I opened it. Inside lay my Silver Star – the medal itself, the battle ribbon for my uniform, the lapel stud for civilian clothes and the official citation, signed by General Krulak, Commander of the Marines in the Western Pacific.

My stomach twisted. Rage welled up in my chest. I threw the box across the room hollering, "You goddamn sons of bitches! You rotten motherfuckers!" Then I realized that nobody was listening, that no one could hear my invectives, which meant they accomplished nothing. So, I went over and picked up the medal, took it and carefully hung it on a loop of sturdy string in my toilet bowl. Every morning after that, I'd urinate on it. This was how I could piss on the U.S. military and all of the politicians. However, the months went by. The pleasure faded. I noticed the ribbon was rotting and the metal star corroding. One morning, before relieving myself, I decided to pull the Silver Star out of the toilet, cleaned it off, and put it away.

I decided to keep it as a reminder of the guys who I lost. I never had a chance to say good-bye. I would never forget them.

Draft Dodgerology

During the Vietnam war, 570,000 young men committed draft violations that could have resulted in prison sentences of up to 5 years. Of these, 210,000 were reported to the U.S. Justice Department for potential prosecution, including over a hundred thousand that had burned their draft cards. About 10,000 cases were brought to trial. Approximately 8,750 were convicted. 3,250 were imprisoned, roughly half for 7-month to 2-year sentences.

During my stay at UCSF, and later at a Kaiser lab, I felt called to duty. As a doctor, I knew I could be saving lives. I personally knew grunts that had been killed unnecessarily. I wanted to do what I could to limit the death toll. I designated myself what I called a Board Certified Draft Dodgerologist. My efforts began with Bill Hawkins, a big black kid who worked as a janitor in our laboratories. Always ready with a cheery good morning for me, Bill was one of the few people who didn't look down on me for being a Vietnam veteran. One morning, though, he came to me with a worried look on his face.

"Doc, I'm gettin' drafted," he told me, in a tone of dismay. "Ain't there some way I can get out?"

"Did you get called for a physical?" I inquired.

"Yeah, Doc. What do I do?"

"Are you sick? Is there anything wrong with you?"

"Not that I can think of. I ain't never been in the hospital," he said, pondering his past, "but only once 'at I c'n think of, and that 'as only the emergency room."

"What was that about?"

"When I was a kid playin' ball and I fell into the bushes and got stung by a bee. I swole up all over – couldn't breathe."

"That's it!" I shouted, recalling an incident at Khe Sanh of anaphylactic shock. "You got bee sting allergy! That should make you 4-F!"

"You mean, Doc, gettin' stung by a lousy bee can get you out of the Army?" he asked, incredulous.

"I think so, man. I think so. Come on into the lab. I'll take a history and do a physical on you. I'll play like I'm your doctor and write a letter saying that this allergy is too serious to allow you to be drafted. When do you have to report?"

"Next week, Doc."

I brought him into my laboratory and performed a cursory history and physical. Other than the episode with the bee sting, I could find nothing really wrong with him. I needed a little stronger evidence before feeling comfortable about writing a letter to the Draft Board, declaring him ineligible.

"Hey, Bill, remember last year when you got stung by a wasp and had trouble breathing?" I asked, winking at him.

"Huh? What'd'ya say, Doc?" Bill was certainly not Phi Beta Kappa, but I felt he was far better than cannon fodder for the defense contractors.

"Bill, you remember when the wasp stung you and you almost died... last year... Remember?" I asked intently.

"Oh yeah, Doc, yeah. Maybe I remember now. Almost forgot," he added sheepishly. "But ain't that lyin', Doc? Ain't that bad?"

"I don't know, man. Is it bad to lie to Nazis or the Ku Klux Klan?"

"No way, brother. No way. Jesus! I almost like to die last year when that wasp bit me. Wow! That was bad, Doc, wasn't it?", with his last words punctuated with bellowing laughter.

"Too bad you're not healthy enough to serve your country in its battle against the yellow scourge."

"What'd ya say, Doc?"

"Nothing. Just keep quiet about this and come back tomorrow. I'll have a letter for you."

"Okay, Doc. I sure hope this works!" strolling off with a worried smile.

That next morning, Bill came to the laboratory and I gave him the letter.

"Be sure you give this to the doctor who gives you the draft physical. Don't give it to a clerk, only a doctor," I insisted. "You bet, brother, you bet," he said, carefully placing the letter in his coat pocket.

One morning several weeks later, Bill came in with a liquor bottle wrapped in a brown paper bag. "Here, Doc. I owe you this, a fifth of black Jack Daniel's whisky."

"They bought it! You're 4-F!" I shouted, hugging him and jumping with glee.

"You bet, man! The Doc took one look at your letter and said, 'You're 4-F, brother.' 4-F means Uncle Sam don't want me. I'm free! I'm free! And it's all 'cause of you," he shouted with tears of joy streaming down his cheeks.

"Thank God," I mumbled.

"What ya say, Doc?"

"Nothin', man, nothin'." I turned back to my lab bench. Of all the life-saving medicine I'd practiced, the case of this young man was the most satisfying and life-changing for me. All of the other boys were already mangled young bodies. Bill was healthy, intact and unscarred, not a what should have been, but what can be. This was true preventive medicine.

I really do have the cure for acute lead poisoning.

It wasn't long before the word spread. I was inundated with young men who were being drafted. There was a sudden epidemic of bee-sting allergies in the community. The Selective Service doctors, usually active-duty draftees, went along with the conspiracy. They were more than happy to have a reason to consider these rejections.

One young man wrote me a short note:

241

"Unfortunately, due to my serious bee sting allergy, Uncle Sam will not allow me to serve my country in its terrible struggle against the wicked forces of evil in Southeast Asia. Thank you for your help."

After about fifty cases, the Draft Board woke up to what was happening. I discovered that pressure being brought to bear on me. My boss, Hugh Fudenberg, called me into his office. "Al, I don't care what your politics are. You're here to do immunology research. Just carry on your political activities after working hours. That will take a lot of pressure off me."

"Who's putting pressure on you?" I inquired.

"The chairman's busting his butt to get funding from the Hughes Medical Foundation. Since they're major defense contractors, the Hughes guys don't like to see anti-war activity, especially in places where they're paying the bills."

"What does Hughes Industries have to do with the chairman of the Department of Medicine and this school?" I wondered out loud.

He quipped with a sardonic tone, "I guess there's more money to be made in medicine than war. This is the beginning of the Health/Industrial Complex, you know." I angrily responded, "They invade everything, even my profession".

You dumped me into a holocaust.
You wasted my buddies and destroyed families.
I lost mine.
Professionally, my reputation has been stained.
And… the IRS is shaking me down.
Go to the hell I've known.
I really wish I were dead.

Chapter Thirteen
Vera My Lover and Life Saver

I tell everybody.

Vera saved my life. Why she stuck with me all these years, I will never know, but I certainly fully appreciate it. I would be dead without her.

The day she passes away is the day I will want to join her.

On June 15, 1971, I was attending the American Association of Immunologists meeting in San Francisco. That is where I met Vera Byers, Ph.D., young and gorgeous, whom I noticed immediately. There she was, reviewing displays in the scientific poster section of the convention.

Physically, Vera was stunning, a former ballet dancer. Intellectually, she was absolutely brilliant, a highly productive scientist with a keen interest in clinical immunology. I was in love instantly. I asked her out, generating what I thought was the clever excuse of talking about our pioneering work in immunology.

At dinner in Sausalito, trying to impress her, I suggested I could teach her a few things, never having ascertained that, in fact, Vera had a PhD in immunology and written 20 papers. Obviously, my attention had been entirely focused on her great legs.

Being so crudely objectified physically and diminished intellectually, Vera abruptly stood up, dumped her bowl of minestrone soup on my head and briskly walked out, leaving me there with everyone at the restaurant aghast. I realized just how smart she was telling me to get lost.

However, I didn't give up.

Vera finally gave in to my vision of foreverness and we began living together.

The Lady and The Tramp

In our early years, without me fully realizing it, Vera had undertaken a seemingly futile project to civilize me. When I first met her, I wasn't a hippie by any means, but I never paid much attention to my dress or demeanor. For my wardrobe I kept three cardboard moving boxes in the bedroom: clean, semi-clean, and dirty. When things got too dirty, I took them to the laundry. I didn't have long hair and I was clean-shaven. But I never paid attention to what I wore.

Pulling from a shopping bag, Vera handed me underwear and then said, "Okay, now you are going to wear these." Then she produced a pair of socks, and I began rebelling. I didn't want to wear socks. It was a pain in the ass to put them on. But I did. Then, a belt. And a turtleneck sweater. Going too far, she broached the subject of a tie – and I got really agitated – "It's just a ribbon you tie around your neck!"

Somebody could choke you.

Of course, when a Vietnam vet said something like that, even joking, everybody got spooked. We looked bad and talked even worse. Later, I found out that people felt uncomfortable, perhaps a bit unsafe around me. So, they left me alone. But they left me out in the cold, too. I never got to the point where I was socially acceptable, although I was making an attempt to assimilate by dressing like everyone else.

Truth be known, Vera still complains about my persistent sloppiness.

Finally Talking Her Into Taking the Leap Again

When this brilliant lady stepped into my world, in all of my brokenness and idiosyncrasies, I began to transform, caring about whether there would be a tomorrow. With her, I wanted one and then another. Inside of me, a healer was being healed.

"We've got to get married." I told her. She'd already been trapped in a bad marriage and acrimonious divorce. She was in no hurry by any means. In order to placate me, however, we went to get the marriage license.

Vera kept on figuring out reasons why not to go through with it. I kept pleading. Enough time had passed that I decided to call City Hall to check on whether the license was still valid. "Yes," I was told. The clerk adding, "And on Tuesdays, the ceremony's free."

Today was it!

Rushing over to Vera in her lab, I proclaimed, "Shut down your work. We're going to get married today. Free of charge!"

'What? Wait! I… I've got to do this important experiment now," she demurred.

I was persistent. "We'll come back and I'll help you finish it."

At City Hall, ascending the staircase slowly and pensively, she stopped. "Wait a minute. Are you sure we're doing the right thing?"

"Hell yes, we're here. Come on, let's just get it done."

Vera was afraid, thinking her life was going away. Here she was, divorced and free, trading one crazy bastard for another. But I got us up there.

Finally, I guess, leaving it to fate, she suggested, "Okay. Now let's flip a coin. Heads we get married, tails we don't."

We had the justice of the peace flip a coin, and it came out heads. Vera lost, so we got hitched. To this day we don't know when it was. It was on a Tuesday, in the spring of 1973. While we've been "happily married ever since," we never celebrate our anniversary because we don't just know when it is.

Establishing Ourselves

Early on in our marriage, Vera received her M.D. from UCSF, having already served on the faculty in immunology there. While in medical school, she continued to be a prolific author, publishing 21 peer reviewed medical journal articles. Simultaneously, I finished my medical training in pediatric immunology and became Board Certified in Clinical Pathology, Allergy Immunology and Emergency Medicine.

I was allowed to take these boards without ever having to work as a resident. Permission to take my exams was granted by Dr. Francis A. Sooy, Chancellor at UCSF Medical School and a fellow flight surgeon who served in the U.S. Naval Medical Corps during World War II. He was an avid pilot who loved restoring and flying his WWII trainer. In 1986, Dr. Sooy was killed as a passenger in a private plane crash in Solano County, California.

At the height of the AIDS crisis, Vera directed Positive Action Healthcare, a clinic in San Francisco. Besides continuing my research in immunology, I worked in emergency rooms. Seeing this older doctor come in to treat them, "Okay", they might say, "We can relax. Obviously, you know what you're doing." I'd shiver without them noticing it. I'd think –

That's what the wounded grunts would tell me.

At least in this modern medical facility, I was presented with much better odds of success.

Unbeknownst to anyone else, I was also relieved by not having to carry any morphine syrettes on my lapel, being routinely tasked with performing euthanasia.

Quest for Cancer's Cure and Victory Over Autoimmune Diseases

Over the decades, both Vera and I joined the fight in the war on cancer. We participated in advancing the emerging field of immunology, being early pioneers in discovering how the immune system works, the role of various immune cells in the human body's arsenal in its war against pathogens, and how that system can malfunction.

Through the years, I've held positions at UCSF including Associate Professor of Immunology. I hold two patents in immunotherapeutic regimens. Together, Vera and I were the first to test the effectiveness of monoclonal antibodies clinically and used RNA in the treatment of osteogenic sarcoma. One of our patients was a young boy who had been stricken with that cancer, which unfortunately required a leg amputation.

As a team, with Vera in the lead, we helped pave the path towards the successful use of TNF Alpha blocker medications, specifically Enbrel, for the treatment of chronic inflammation and autoimmune diseases like Rheumatoid Arthritis, Crohn's Disease and Ulcerative Colitis. Over the years, Vera and I have drawn our own blood countless times for use in research testing.

"We needed some. No one else was around to donate it. So, it's Vera or me. Or both." I've often commented.

Rewards of Research in Pediatric Immunology

During my work at UCSF in pediatric immunology, one of my first patients was Johnny Perez, who suffered from the obscure Wiskott-Aldridge syndrome, a congenital immunodeficiency which, up until then, had been untreatable and uniformly fatal in young children.

At that time, I had been talking with one of my colleagues, Dr. Lynn Spitler, about one of her pet projects. It was a transfer factor – a low molecular weight immune modulator derived from human lymphocytes and shown able to passively transfer skin test reactivity from an immune donor to a naive recipient.

Can this be a breakthrough? Such quests always thrilled me.

What this work involves is taking minute amounts of material from immune persons and giving it to non-immune persons, immunity can be transferred from one person to another in that process.

As I began evaluating Johnny, I realized that transfer factor might be therapeutically beneficial for children who did not have immune competence. Mentioning my idea to Lynn, using transfer factor therapeutically in the treatment of a child with a congenital immunodeficiency disorder, her initial reaction was negative. In fact, she screamed and hollered: "You can't do that! It's unethical! It's never been used in a treatment before. How can you possibly think of using that on such a defenseless child?"

My response was, "The child's going to die anyway. Why not try it? It seems to be reasonably innocuous." After protracted sparring back and forth, my point of view prevailed. We were successful in altering his immune deficiency disorder. We were able to render him infection-free for over one year. During the heady period of this success, we elected to try transfer factor on other diseases.

During the onset of my research, through a friend, I encountered a young girl with incurable osteogenic sarcoma – bone cancer. Emotionally distraught, my friend began crying. "I wish there was something we could give her to make the tumor melt away."

Bingo! A light went on in my head. What if I could "make the tumor melt away!" Because osteogenic sarcoma appeared to be caused by a virus, it was totally reasonable to presume that we could boost the child's immune reactivity to this viral element and perhaps help her get better. To treat her, I immediately went about the task of developing transfer factor from members of her household.

This girl had a quite large tumor in her pelvis which had been extensively irradiated. While the radiation therapy was going on, we collected blood from her parents and her older sister and extracted transfer factor from the white blood cells of these donors. When the radiation was completed, we began the transfer factor therapy. The initial treatments went without a hitch. In fact, there appeared to be a significant reduction in the size of the tumor mass over and above what would be expected from the radiation alone.

We were all excited.

When we started the treatment, I gave her one in a trillion chances of surviving the tumor. Now we had significant improvement, so I gave her one in a million chance. Unfortunately, after the first blush of success, the tumor began to grow, and the child passed away.

This promising original work gave us considerable insight into tumor immunology. We got funding, too. With an NIH grant to study transfer factor immunotherapy in cancer, we took on seventeen more young bone cancer patients. Because the tumor had a 95% death rate after diagnosis, only one of those seventeen could be expected to be alive five years.

As a result of our treatment, however, today sixteen of these then-children are adults who are alive and well.

Redemption Always on the Horizon

Is it possible for a wretched human being like myself to find redemption?

The gift of my surviving the decades after the Vietnam war meant returning to that original dream. I wanted to share what abilities were bestowed upon me in the field of pediatric medicine and cancer research – turning my efforts to killing a killer.

That scrappy kid from the West Chicago ghetto had survived and so had that pediatric cancer doctor. And, he actually flourished. In that war against fatal disease, I was the second author of the first research paper describing the critical role of T-cells in the immune system, which fight infection and cellular dysfunction that leads to cancer and other diseases.

In 1970 at UCSF, I was part of a team which was the first to use MRNA in humans, teaching our cells how to create a protein that triggers an immune response. Fifty years later, that break-through in medical science, as we now know, led us to the creation of vaccines to combat the COVID-19 pandemic.

For my role in the advancement of medical science, however, I was always treated as an outcast, an oddball, a lunatic and a real quack,

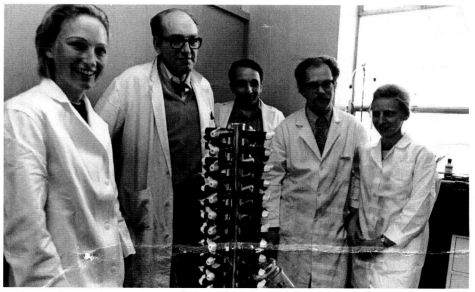

Early 1970's UCSF immunology research team and its groundbreaking breakthroughs in mRNA technology, leading to creation of life-saving vaccines. In center of photo is Al Levin, M.D (Credit: USCF)

however brilliant in birthing precognitions of future advances in the cure and treatment of life-threatening diseases.

I had atoned, but I guess I never fully extended the graces of empathy and understanding.

Chapter Fourteen
Never Ended For Us

"The 'lucky' ones got shipped home. Their tours of duty ended. The 'unlucky' got maimed. The 'luckiest' got killed."
Unknown Author

When I returned home from Vietnam, I was not the same. I never would be. For a time, I was envious of those who died. They were at peace. I never have been. I doubt I'll ever be in this life. I have no idea what is ahead.

I just appreciate what is.

Coming back to America, I was not the bright-eyed idealist with his head in the clouds. No longer a dreamer. No longer an innocent with the world at his fingertips. No longer did people smile at my bright, shiny eyes and my rosy cheeks. No longer would any benevolent mentor take me under his wing to nurture my budding career in academic medicine. My mood was now intense, my actions abrupt and jerky. I tended to repel the more squeamish. People found themselves repulsed by the intense, beady stare coming from my deep-set eyes framed by the sunken cheeks of my hawk-like face. People knew to fear my anger. That rage that seethed inside of me which spawned a U.S. government-trained killer. Was I psychopathic? Most of us were. You'd almost have to be. You're capable of throwing a switch inside your head into the mode of kill or be killed. Coming home, how does a combat warrior just return to who he was?

Albeit disgracefully, the Vietnam war ended. But was the conflict over for all of us?

If you're old enough, you remember witnessing the fall of Saigon on television. Or you've seen the grainy newsreel footage of masses of people, our collaborators and friends, trying to escape, fearing deadly reprisals. They rushed the U.S. embassy gates, climbing the walls, scaling rooftops, attempting to board outgoing helicopter flights.

251

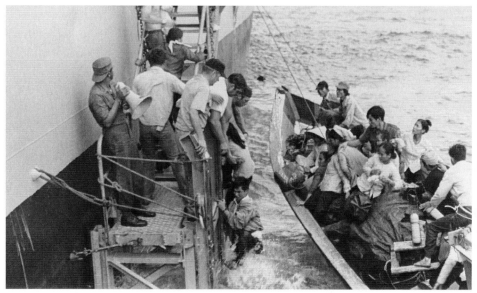

Refugees from the Phan Rang area board the USS Durham (LKA-114) from small craft, to be transferred to a safer area, 3 April 1975 (Source: National Archives)

Such scenes of utter desperation again unfolded before us when the U.S. retreated following 20 years of warfare in Afghanistan. The country fell back in the hands of the Taliban in just over a week.

Back in 1968, we listened to Walter Cronkite, a stalwart of TV News broadcasting, in his editorial about the Vietnam conflict –

"For it seems now more certain than ever, that the bloody experience of Vietnam is to end in a stalemate. To say that we are closer to victory today is to believe in the face of the evidence, the optimists who have been wrong in the past."
Walter Cronkite
Editorial
February 27, 1968

Even with such a bleak, but realistic forecast for the outcome of the war, we continued fighting for years. Then we pulled out, like others had. Our leaders here certainly were never going to stop lying about why we went and then just gave up in a stalemate. Tens of thousands of us were killed. Hundreds of thousands were physically and mentally damaged or destroyed.

For what?

At the end of his TV News broadcasts, Cronkite famously signed out with, "And, that's the way it is."

252

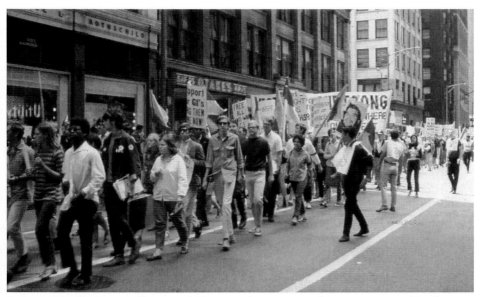

Protesters in the Streets of New York City marching against the Vietnam War (Credit: David Wilson)

Was that way it was? Was the war over, just like that?

Perhaps, for others. Not for us.

We came home to spit and tomatoes – verbal assaults and vile insults. Our vets were treated as outcasts and derelicts.

Junk Mules

A lot of us came home addicted to heroin. When we landed in Southeast Asia, U.S. soldiers were a perfect market for the heroin trade, which the CIA was supporting, as explained to me during my involvement in covert operations. This popular but highly addictive drug had been recently refined in cartel-controlled clandestine labs to a remarkably increased potency of 90 to 95% purity. Many of our vets not only got hooked, but also were involved in trafficking this highly lucrative narcotic, both amongst themselves and transporting it back home.

I never touched any of it.

Thank You for Your Service

These days, military veterans get recognition. Active duty vets board the airplane first. They are openly thanked for their service. I could put on my military uniform now and attend veterans' parades or participate in Honor Flights, where vets are flown at no cost to Washington D.C. to visit the memorials built in their honor.

I don't have a uniform and I haven't attended any events. If they help my fellow vets, I'm happy for them. Perhaps all of these patriotic efforts somehow help America relieve its collective guilt for sending us?

No Military Uniform in My Closet

If I were to assemble my uniform, you probably first notice my rank – Lieutenant. Yep, I was never promoted. In fact, I was threatened three times with court-martial. But then, as you have come to understand, they probably thought, "Shit, what other dumbass can we find to take his place? Forget it, send him back. He'll probably get killed anyway and be out of our hair for good."

Send me back, they did. Get killed? Somehow not.

However, looking at my uniform, without knowing any of that, perhaps you'd then notice the Naval Aviation insignia and recognize the commendations: Silver Star, Bronze Star with Combat "V" Valor, Combat Action Ribbon and an Air Medal with 3 Gold Stars.

Just looking at those, understanding what they mean, you might think, "Wow."

Perhaps you've been told it was the uniform of the most decorated flight surgeon in the Vietnam War. Your reverential response might be, "There's a true hero right there."

Imagine then, if you actually met me, and told me that, in a genuinely respectful manner. I'd cringe and quietly get irritated, and perhaps, seethe with a little hostility. Not that I mean harm. But the anger overtakes me. I want to scream and cry, naming the real heroes I knew who gave their everything. My life continued, as tumultuous as it was. Theirs didn't. To this day, I am overwhelmed at times with profound sadness and despondency.

I hate what America did to us, but especially to them.

I do find comfort and healing in attending our USMC aviation squadron reunions. No pomp. No circumstance. With these old farts, I can genuinely relate. We lived it together. We survived it. We remember those who didn't. And, those who made it home from the war, but no longer remain with us, except in our thoughts.

Our memories of lost buddies remain steadfast. At least, as long as we still have functioning memories from which to draw. It's like the guy who goes to the doctor and says "Doctor, I'm having memory problems." The doctor questions, "When did that happen?" The guy pauses and then asks, "When did what happen?"

I'll continue to go as long as I can. It's always been and continues to be a great group of guys.

My Dogs

What recovery I have experienced since my Vietnam days is primarily due to Vera's support and inspiration, but also, of course, what my dogs so genuinely provide me. We've always had them. We like big dogs – German Shepherd mixes, Collies, Borzoi and Lurchers. Right now, running my household and often occupying our king-size bed are Raffels, a Labradoodle, Labrador/Standard Poodle mix and Clarissa, a Whippet/Poodle mix. They know us both so well.

They love us, unconditionally. We love them back. They insist that you join them in the now, when it's time to eat, for a snuggle or some exercise. Looking at you eye to eye, they are quite demanding and persuasive, but sweetly so.

Let's enjoy! Indulgences await!

Admittedly, our dogs are fat and certainly spoiled. In the back of our car is a giant bed for them, where they travel in comfort. They occupy our laps on the couch. They lay at our feet while we pound away at our keyboards. Walking the steep hills in our neighborhood, they keep us fit. Emotionally, they keep us alive. These precious creatures offer so freely their warm and genuine affection.

We return it joyfully.

Taking to the Skies

While our careers soared, so did we. I was already an aviator. Vera got her private pilot's license and attained an instrument rating. We bought an airplane, and later, a faster one. We loved our Piper Malibu. Nothing like the freedom of flight or the spectacular sunsets

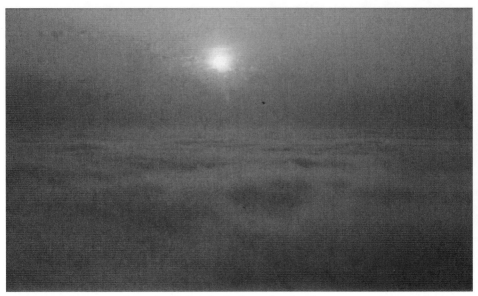

The view of the sunset from the cockpit high above the clouds is never tiring (Credit: Dave Petteys)

in the heights above.

Not A Day Passes

Now, I'm old. I'm in my eighties. I'm not flying around like I used to. I know I'm counting the days. But I've always deeply appreciated how I was given a chance to live my life. My close buddies and the countless numbers of nameless faces of fellow Marines that I still remember in Vietnam were not afforded that opportunity.

Triggers

For those of us who survived, the war continued to rage within us. My day could be going just fine. Then, out of nowhere, a powerful trigger occurs. Something simple can do it. A loud noise. A certain smell. That sheer panic and fear grip you. Your chest tightens, as if being placed in a vice. You heart rate accelerates. Negative emotions overwhelm you and sweep you away as if by torrential floodwaters.

For me, fireworks on the Fourth of July bring on the worst moments. I find a dark place. I curl up and I break down into tears. Of course, now, I admit it's not so bad. I've lost most of my hearing due to the repeated damage to my ear drums from my combat experience.

My poor wife has to yell at me to get my attention when I forget to put my hearing aids in or their batteries are low.

PTSD

Through the ages, following wars, returning combat vets have always suffered from Post Traumatic Stress Disorder. We've called it by various names: Combat Fatigue, Shell Shock, War Neurosis, PTSD and, interestingly, Soldier's Heart, which is a Civil War term describing an increased propensity among combat veterans for cardiovascular disease. This brutal disorder produces nightmares or intrusive, unwanted memories, anxiety and depression.

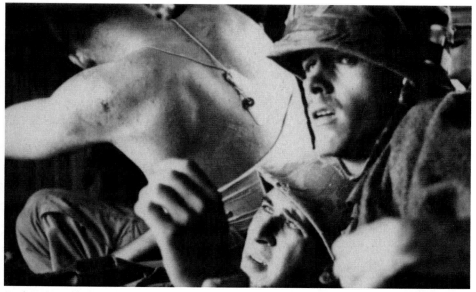

Re-living combat experiences plagues the veterans who survive to return home (Credit: USMC)

Yes, war vets do return to their lives, to a job and a family, or attempt to do so, but suffer from war-related disabilities and early demise.

To deal with it, we shut down. I did. I still do. We turn to drugs and alcohol. I drink Jack Daniels every night to sleep. We can't always control our anger and rage. We lose our wives and alienate our children. We get fired from jobs or held back from advancing a career.

Quoting the book, *Working Class War – American Combat Soldiers and Vietnam* by Christian Appy, "Society as a whole was certainly unable and unwilling to receive these men with the support and understanding they needed." Appy goes on: "The most common experiences of rejection were not explicit acts of hostility but quieter, sometimes more devastating forms of withdrawal, suspicion, and indifference. The feeling toward them was, 'Stay away – don't contaminate us with whatever you've brought back from Vietnam.'"

Studies estimate that an estimated 800,000 Vietnam veterans suffered from Post Traumatic Stress Disorder. Those are actual diagnoses. Countless others suffered in silence, and still do.

However, the VA didn't even admit that this illness existed until years later. And benefits? We were offered $200 a month.

We felt isolated and alone. Our anger was only exacerbated. There is no doubt as to why a lot of us, an estimated 25%, ended up incarcerated.

Our struggles back home were not a dystopia. They are real and persistent.

Switching the Battle to the Courtroom

In 1995, I became a lawyer, attending Golden Gate University and being admitted to practice in California, Texas and Nevada. Academics were always my forte with my score on the Texas bar examination being the 4th all-time highest ever in that state.

Healing and now advocating, I discovered, were in my blood.

As a medical expert, then as a trial attorney, I focused on toxic tort cases. One of my court battles was against Dow Chemical Company involving Agent Orange, the defoliant sprayed throughout Vietnam to kill the vegetation where the enemy might be hiding. They sprayed it on the battlefields, along the perimeter of our bases, the quarters, runways and around landing zones.

Beginning in the early 1960s, the U.S. began conducting these herbicide spraying operations. President Kennedy authorized Operation Ranch-Hand, the codename for the U.S. Air Force program. From 1962-71, for nine years, the U.S. military sprayed over an estimated 20 million gallons of the so-called "rainbow herbicides" in Vietnam, Laos and Cambodia. It is estimated that over 2 million U.S. service members were exposed to these potentially toxic defoliants.

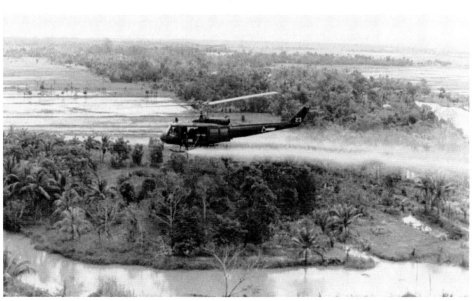

UH-1 sprays Agent Orange across the rural Vietnamese landscape, decimating animal and plant life (Credit: U.S. Army)

Known as Agent Orange, due to the orange bands on the storage drums, the product itself was white and powder-like. It was sprayed, appearing like snowfall, from helicopters and low-flying C-123 Provider aircraft. It did its job, laying bare broad swaths of once lush landscape.

This defoliant can be harmless, if contaminants, specifically dioxin, are removed. Dioxin is a known carcinogen and remains in the environment for decades, perhaps centuries, impacting the food chain and posing a hazard to people and animals.

Unbeknownst to us, the Agent Orange dumped in the Southeast Asia conflict was the cheaper version, the type where the dioxin was not removed. It could have been made safe. In fact, in the U.S., the contaminated version was banned. Only sales of the decontaminated product were allowed.

But they dumped the poison on us, just to save a few bucks.

As you would expect, in the years and decades since returning home, Vietnam vets were stricken with cancers and their children were born with defects related to Agent Orange exposure, particularly spina bifida.

In Vietnam, we were not warned. We weren't told of the threat to our health and that of our offspring. We were not protected. Again, we were an expendable bunch of stupid and gullible grunts.

Warnings?

None whatsoever.

We didn't know.

Now, knowing these facts, if this didn't upset jurors, nothing would.

Hey, Dow.

There were potential bogies on your radar.

Gigantic judgments could be forthcoming, once the evidence of corporate conscious indifference and profiteering in these cases was presented in trial. But, litigation is risky and expensive. Even with winning a huge verdict, could it eventually be collected? Any jury awards would surely be appealed to the higher courts which are more sympathetic to corporate interests.

But, we were angry. We were committed. We fought... and lost.

As an expert, I argued that dioxin exposure causes cancer. I was accused of being a junk scientist. On Dow's payroll were experts, hired by the defendants, who got on the stand under oath and testified that dioxin didn't cause cancer. That was not true. But, of course, they were paid handsomely for their opinions.

It reminds me of the CEOs of all the leading cigarette companies who claimed smoking their products didn't cause cancer. They funded studies making such assertions and held them up as evidence that they held no responsibility for the millions of smoking-related deaths worldwide.

In the Agent Orange case, overseen by Jack Weinstein, a Brooklyn federal judge, experts testifying for the stricken vets and their disabled children, who linked dioxin exposure to their illnesses, were disqualified. Quoting Judge Weinstein, a Navy WWII vet who served aboard the USS Jallao submarine, "An expert can be found to testify to the truth of almost any theory, no matter how frivolous." In dismissing the case, the judge cited grounds that the use of the herbicide in warfare had been legal under international law at the time.

Today, the VA recognizes that exposure to Agent Orange or other herbicides during military service is the probable cause of numerous types of cancer in Vietnam veterans including Chronic B-Cell leukemias, Hodgkin Lymphoma, Non-Hodgkin Lymphoma, Multiple Myeloma, prostate cancer and respiratory cancers.

I was ridiculed at the time, labeled a crazed junk scientist. However, I was absolutely right.

A Paltry Effort to Help Those Who Served You

Confronted with what they knew but not wanting to risk it being revealed, Dow did put an end to the court battle. It settled the class action lawsuit, agreeing to pay a paltry $197 million in cash payments on 105,000 claims, averaging about $3800 per claimant. Other limited funding was provided by Dow to relevant social service organizations. In exchange, the U.S. Congress passed legislation granting Dow Chemical immunity from any further related civil liabilities.

As always, it was about shareholder equity, executive golden parachutes and pocket-lined politicians. We were just the gullible and compliant, so easily brainwashed.

They owned us in Vietnam. We did their dirty work. Then they basically abandoned us.

Lost Time

When Vietnam vets came back to America, those who survived and overcame the steep obstacles that faced us, we grew to treasure time, which is the most precious of all that we possess. It's really all we have.

From what we witnessed so horrifically in our war experiences, we became painfully aware of the fact that no one can know how much time is allotted to us in our lifetimes. You are here. Then, you are gone. As I've been granted the privilege and opportunity to grow into old age, I've gained greater respect and appreciation for each tick of the clock that I am able to experience and share with those around me.

Most Vietnam vets, I realize, came out of the war and moved forward. Many have died pre-maturely since they returned. We did rise up as we were able and keep going, but we are still battling: to maintain our sanity, to overcome physical and mental obstacles, and discover coping tools that enable us to manage and accomplish what we had always hoped we could.

I was able to succeed because I discovered that I am not alone.

My wife is with me, along with my friends and community. Frankly, Jack Daniels is one of my most helpful companions. He helps get me to sleep and keeps the nightmares in quiescence. As Vietnam vets, we lost out for years on therapy for our PTSD and many of us turned to drugs and alcohol to deal with our daily demands and struggles.

When the bad dreams do return to haunt me, they're always the same – helicopter explosions, seeing comrades burned to death. In my nightmares, I'm not just re-creating images of actual events in my mind, I am jolted awake re-living them. My guts wrench. The nausea returns. I vomit, while the tears flow uncontrollably.

I wish I couldn't remember. But I can never forget.

The Wall

A few years ago, I made a personal and private visit to the Vietnam Memorial, or "The Wall" as it's called, located in Washington D.C. It was designed by Maya Lin, a Yale architectural student and is constructed of granite panels in a "V" shape, with one end pointing towards Lincoln Memorial and the other towards the Washington Monument.

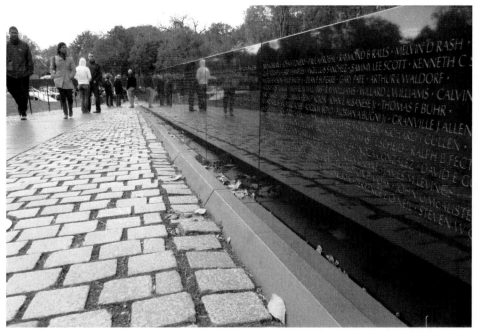

Known simply as "The Wall", the Vietnam Memorial in Washington D.C. remains a site of active grieving by surviving comrades and loved ones (Source: Wikimedia Commons)

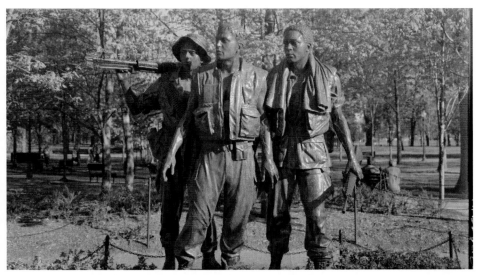

Located by the Vietnam Memorial, the Three Soldiers bronze statute by Frederick Hart was created to portray the broad ethnic make-up of U.S. troops in the Vietnam conflict (Source: U.S. National Park Service)

Etched on the wall are the names of the killed or missing in action. As of 2021, there are 58,281 names, listed according to date of death or disappearance. They appear with the buddies who were lost alongside them. The 400-foot memorial symbolizes for our nation, a deep scar that's been cut in the ground. Visiting the site are those who continue to actively grieve their losses.

Nearby are statutes of fellow combat soldiers and female nurses.

Being able to actually reach out and physically touch a name on this wall is a healing experience – to make contact with those who did not come home with their comrades, to their loved ones, their parents, grandparents, their spouses, children, professions, churches and local communities. Here those left behind have an opportunity to pay their respects and continue to process the sorrow surrounding their losses.

I went there when I didn't really want to. Doing this would be terribly painful, I knew. I was not even sure if I would able to approach the wall once I got there. I endured this trip for a solitary reason – to visit Stan Lewis and the others. In my hand, I had an old metal lighter my corpsmen gave to me.

On the front is inscribed "To: Bac Si Al Levin" and on the back "It sucks. From: The Snuffys Gary Panko, Sean Barry, Paul Fitzgerald, Dan Sullivan, Bill Sperb and Fred Newcomb."

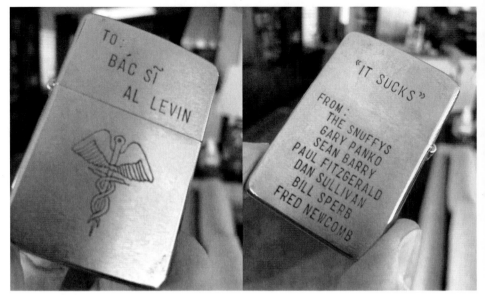

The inscribed metal lighter given to Dr. Al Levin by fellow Marine comrades (Source: J.B. Gentry)

Bac Si means doctor in Vietnamese. About the war, I always said "It sucks." And Snuffys is a Navy term, referring to low ranking enlisted men. From that group of my corpsmen, Gary was the only survivor and later died by suicide.

I went the wall to talk to all of my guys…

You're the reason I lived.

You didn't deserve to die. You were lied to. So was I.

They said I would like you. They were wrong. I love you.

And, I miss you.

My memories of them remain steadfast. I jest about someday sinking into the nothingness of dementia, if my tattered body doesn't give out before my brain. To this day, I continue to work on research into treating and possibly curing Alzheimer's Disease through the long term use of anti-inflammatory medications.

As long as I can function, to think and to breathe, I will strive to fulfill my commitment to remain present for my buddies who couldn't. In the aftermath of my horrific experiences and past actions, I became better able to empathize with others, especially with my patients who suffer profound losses. My enhanced awareness and compassion for those in pain made me a better physician.

It made me better human being.

Epilogue

$6.5 trillion dollars

That's an official estimate of what we'll have spent since 9/11 fighting proxy wars in the Middle East and Asia – $2.2 trillion upfront and the interest continues to mount into what will become an astronomically huge pile of debt. Unlike previous wars, in the 20 years we've spent fighting in Iraq and Afghanistan, funding came from supplemental appropriations. Basically, we printed the money and then borrowed it, so a lot of the financial burden, paying for these wars, will fall on future generations. That's an almost incomprehensible outflow of taxpayer dollars, about twenty grand for every man, women and child in our country, a string of one-hundred dollar bills that would make 25 rings around the planet, or over dozen trips to the Moon and back.

Additionally, there is the immeasurable cost in human lives. In recent wars, seven thousand U.S. service members and contractors killed. Hundreds of thousands more were maimed, physically and mentally.

And who gained, as a result of these conflicts? Back in Vietnam, having acquired Brown and Root in the early 1960s, Halliburton collected hundreds of millions of dollars. As a war profiteer, in recent decades, it collected a total that exceeded a reported $51 billion from the Iraq and Afghanistan wars.

$800+ billion dollars

That's currently the amount of annual revenue flowing into American's military industrial complex. It does employ a couple of million people and there's about a hundred billion in the export of military weaponry.

Hard to comprehend, I know. If we were to match that amount of money, we could raise salaries for every teacher in American to over $200,000 a year. Imagine an educational system with that level of financial commitment to our future.

Where Are the Vietnam Vets Now?

And in human cost? Looking to the Vietnam vets, in 2000, of the 2,709,918 Americans who served in the war, 1,002,511 were still alive. That means roughly 63% died before the age of 53 years old. We are a dying breed. A lot of us died of self-inflicted causes – alcohol, drugs, mishaps, and suicide.

War Is a Racket

In 1935, Major General Smedley D. Butler, a highly decorated U.S. Marine Corps Commanding General, was alarmed. He published *War Is a Racket*, a short book, and conducted a lecture series. America had gotten involved in World War I at great cost to our country and he had witnessed first-hand the greed flourishing around him at our enormous expense. As a teenaged U.S. Marine Corps enlistee, he fought in the Spanish-American War, the Philippine-American War, The Boxer Rebellion in China, the Banana Wars the, Battle for Veracruz during their civil war, and the Haitian invasion following a Presidential assassination. Following a non-combat role in World War I, he became Commanding General at the Marine Corps Base in Quantico, Virginia. General Butler took a leave of absence from the military and became the Philadelphia Director of Public Safety and immediately cracked down on organized crime, beginning his first days on the job closing hundreds of speakeasies. In 1926, he returned to active Marine Corps duty as Commanding General of the Marine Corps base in San Diego. In World War II, General Butler commanded a defense sector. At the time of his retirement, he was the most highly decorated U.S. Marine in its history, having been twice awarded the Congressional Medal of Honor for his exemplary bravery in the U.S. military invasions of Mexico and Haiti. He wrote:
"I wouldn't go to war again as I have done to protect some lousy investment of the bankers. There are only two things we should fight for. One is the defense of our homes and the other is the Bill of Rights. War for

any other reason is simply a racket.

But war-time profits – ah! that is another matter – twenty, sixty, one hundred, three hundred, and even eighteen hundred per cent – the sky is the limit. All that traffic will bear. Uncle Sam has the money. Let's get it.

How many of these war millionaires shouldered a rifle? How many of them dug a trench? How many of them knew what it meant to go hungry in a rat-infested dug-out? How many of them spent sleepless, frightened nights, ducking shells and shrapnel and machine gun bullets? How many of them parried a bayonet thrust of an enemy? How many of them were wounded or killed in battle?

The general public shoulders the bill. Newly placed gravestones. Mangled bodies. Shattered minds. Broken hearts and homes. Economic instability. Depression and all its attendant miseries. Back-breaking taxation for generations and generations."

Beware of Military Industrial Complex

We were further warned 60+ years ago in President Dwight D. Eisenhower's farewell address. Our 34th President, who rose to the rank of 5-star general serving in World War II as the Supreme Commander of the Allied Expeditionary Force in Europe and who led the D-Day invasion, stated in a live national television broadcast:

"We have been compelled to create a permanent armaments industry of vast proportions.

In the councils of government, we must guard against the acquisition of unwarranted influence, whether sought or unsought, by the military-industrial complex. The potential for the disastrous rise of misplaced power exists and will persist.

We must never let the weight of this combination endanger our liberties or democratic processes. We should take nothing for granted. Only an alert and knowledgeable citizenry can compel the proper meshing of the huge industrial and military machinery of defense with our peaceful methods and goals, so that security and liberty may prosper together."

President Dwight D. Eisenhower
Farewell Speech
January 17, 1961

Looking at our future, we have formidable enemies. We are seeing now technological weaponry that operates itself with artificial intelligence. Bullets. Bombs. Rockets. Missiles. Now drones and lasers. Even kamikaze drones. How much more violent will our communities, nations and world be in the future? Where is the next war we will fight? Who will it be? What happens when we begin employing this advanced weaponry against one another? Or, these deadly devices fall into the hands of terrorists? Do we not have enough threats to our existence that our children, grandchildren, great-grandchildren will face and need to overcome?

Training to Kill

We flood our community with deadly weapons, which have turned our homes, schools, public venues and neighborhoods into domestic war zones. Bullets flying. Innocents dying. Making matters more perilous, we are training our kids, primarily our boys, to shoot and kill. We put controllers to violent first-person shooter video games in their hands. One of the most popular, "Counter-Strike" has sold over 25 million units.

In recent years, the U.S. military has used and encouraged many of its soldiers to play these video games as a means to improve combat training. An Iraq War veteran described them as "the ultimate first-person shooter experience ever" and "intensive and highly realistic approaches to tactical combat. The choice of attacking with stealth or unleashing an all-out frontal assault full of mayhem is yours. It's violent, it's chaotic, it's beautiful."

After the 1998 school shooting in Jonesboro, Arkansas, where two 11-year-olds gunned down a teacher and four students, the head of the American Academy of Pediatrics Task Force on Juvenile Violence reminded parents that normal people aren't natural killers. It is a learned skill, derived from abuse and violence in the home and from violence as entertainment in television, the movies and video games.

Should we be concerned, even troubled by the fact that when children play interactive point-and-shoot video games, we are conditioning them to expertly execute these exact motor and reflex skills?

In the future, do we continue training, heavily arming and sending our young adults to fight proxy wars overseas to stalemates or withdrawals, profiting only huge multi-national corporations? Do we continue to destroy countless lives and families, or profoundly damage them?

Aftermath of Our Proxy Wars

Fueling my anger and revulsion are the lies that we've been told and continue to be magnified over and over about why we go to war, extending conflicts for decades, occupying countries until we just leave. Just like Vietnam, many combat vets returning from Iraq, Afghanistan and other conflicts in those regions are severely disabled and disillusioned, especially those who were deployed multiple times. Studies estimate that 40% of combat vets from these conflicts suffer from PTSD and other war-related disabilities. That's more than World War II, Korea and Vietnam combined.

Thus, the demand for medical care, disability compensation and other benefits are astronomical, not just because health care costs have increased and injuries are more severe, but due to medical advances and survival rates. Studies reveal that overall medical care costs could reach at least $2.5 trillion dollars.

Among those combat vets who did survive to return home, suicide, addiction rates and incidents of domestic violence are believed to be underreported. Others argue otherwise. In a Brown University study, as part of the Costs of War project, it concluded that four times as many veterans of the post 9/11 wars have died by suicide than in combat.

"The wounds of this generation are deep," said Peter D. Feaver, a professor of political science at Duke University. "We should not pretend they are not. These are the same issues the Greatest Generation had to wrestle with, and what we have learned is that even wounded people can accomplish a great deal."

Reflecting on my experiences and writing this book was quite difficult for me. Reliving it was extremely disturbing. And I still weep, at times uncontrollably, over the loss of my dear brothers in arms. It still fills me with rage and horror that I must struggle to suppress. However, I also appreciate where through a true life partner, I managed to accomplish what I dreamed of doing, in medical research for the benefit of humanity.

As a physician and combat veteran, I want my legacy to be not that of a war hero, but an anti-proxy war hero. Warfare is not glorious, like in the movies or video games, but quite the opposite. I trust you gain a clearer awareness of that reality from absorbing what I've tried to share from the research I've done and personal memories I possess.

For future generations, my heart-felt message is that in war, nobody really ever wins. Everyone just loses, except for those that made a buck or more.

References

Fire in the Lake
Frances FitzGerald
1972

War Is A Racket
General Smedley D. Butler
1935

Bonnie Sue: A Marine Corps Helicopter Squadron in Vietnam
Marion F. Sturkey
1997

Marine Helo: Helicopter War in Vietnam
David M. Petteys
1995

Masters of the War
A Fighting Marine's Memoir of Vietnam
Ronald E. Winter
2005

U.S. Marines in Vietnam
Major Gary L. Telfer, USMC
Lt. Col. Lane Robers, USMC
V. Keith Fleming, Jr.
USMC History and Museums Division
1984

The End of the Line: The Siege of Khe Sanh
Robert Pisor
2002

Hill Fights
The First Battle of Khe Sahn
Colonel Rod Andrew, Jr. USMC Reserve
Marine Corps University
2017

Working Class War: American Soldiers in Vietnam
Christian G. Appy
1993

A Great Place to Have a War
America in Laos and the Birth of a Military CIA
Joshua Kurlantzick
2017

American War Machine
Peter Dale Scott
2010

Military Spending – 20 Companies Profiting Most from War
Samuel Stebbins
Evan Comen
USA Today
2019

Understanding the Vietnam War Machine
Diana Roose
NARMIC Public Accountability Initiative
2021

Halliburton Deals Recall Vietnam-Era Controversy
John Burnett
NPR
2003

Nixon Prolonged Vietnam War for Political Gain
Colin Schultz
Smithsonian Magazine
2013

Did the M16 Totally Fail During the Vietnam War?
Kyle Mizokami
The National Interest
2018

The Politics of Heroin in Southeast Asia
Alfred W. McCoy
1972

How Drug Dealers Used the U.S. Military to Smuggle Heroin
Blake Stillwell
Insider
2018

The Wretched of the Earth
Frantz Fanon
1961

Free in the Forest: Ethnohistory of Vietnamese Central Highlands
Gerald Cannon Hickey
1976

Should We Have War Crime Trials?
Neil Sheenan
New York Times
1971

On Killing: The Psychological Cost of Learning to Kill in War and Society
Lt. Col. Dave Grossman (Ret.)
1996

The Impact of Killing – How to Prepare the Soldier
Jim Dooley
PBS-Frontline
2005

How Soldiers Deal with the Job of Killing
Stephen Evans
BBC News
2011

A Bulletproof Mind
Peter Maass
New York Times Magazine
2002

Killing in War Leaves Veterans with Lasting Psychological Scars
Laura Kurtzman
UCSF
2016

The Long War Dead
Poems from Vietnam War
Bryan Alec Floyd
1976

Violent Video Games to Train Soldiers
Scott Nicholas Romaniuk and Tobias Burgers
Business Standard
2017

Stop Teaching Our Kids to Kill: A Call to Action Against Video Game Violence
Lt. Col. Dave Grossman (Ret.)
Gloria DeGaetano
1999

In Last Decade, U.S. Veteran Suicides Top Vietnam War Fatalities
Mike Schindler
Military Wire
2020

A Great Place to Have a War: America in Laos and the Birth of a Military CIA
Joshua Kurlantzick
2017

Americans Owe $6.5 Trillion for Wars in Iraq and Afghanistan – And That's Just Interest
CBS News
2021

Veterans Struggle with Issues that Are Often Invisible to Others
Jennifer Steinhauer
New York Times
2021

Air America
Christopher Robbins
1979
Orion Publishing Group

Made in United States
North Haven, CT
04 May 2022

18883271R00161